INDEX

When acne attacks

WHEN ACNE
ATTACKS

EESHTA BHATT
WITH
DR. PARUL KHOT

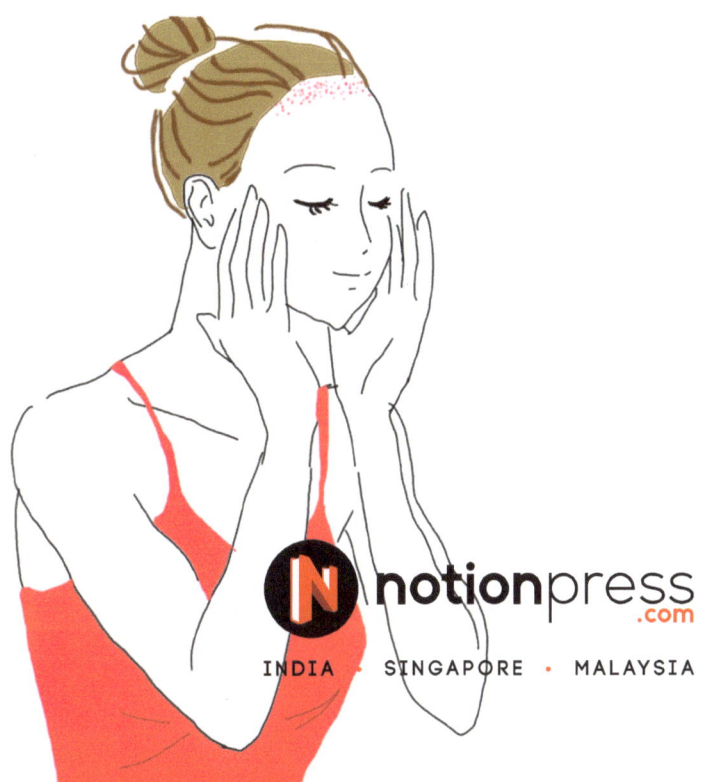

notionpress
.com

INDIA · SINGAPORE · MALAYSIA

Notion Press

No.8, 3rd Cross Street,
CIT Colony, Mylapore,
Chennai, Tamil Nadu – 600004

First Published by Notion Press 2020
Copyright © Eeshta Bhatt 2020
All Rights Reserved.

ISBN 978-1-63714-561-6

Prologue: Opening up about acne

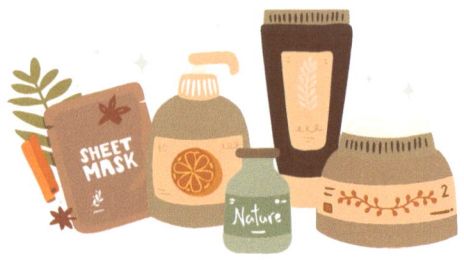

When I was 11 years old, at odds with my mother, experiencing my first breakout, I could imagine nothing worse. Until then, I'd only had to deal with an odd spot or so, that would fade away, no concern for the little hellion I was, running around climbing trees and jumping into dirt puddles.

But suddenly, waking up one day in the summer holidays, my forehead an angry eruption of white-faced pimples, I was led with instant dread at the prospect of starting 6th grade with acne. I was enraged and devastated that I was the only one of my friends suffering in such a manner.

It seems strange to look back on it now, and yet I was incredibly anxious about having to wash my face throughout the school day, carrying around my specific medicated face wash, controlling my diet, and just having to think three times before every action, including staying out in the sun.

The truth of the matter is that I was terrified at what others might think of me.

Public perception was never something I was great at shaking off. Hence, my acne struggles were always at the forefront of my mind; my anxiety playing up whenever anyone looked at my skin a moment too long.

The next years were filled with quarrels with my mother, arguments over being made to drink spinach soup, papaya, limiting takeout, and visiting several dermatologists. Each of whom gave me a range of medications, from antibiotics to ointments, gels, and cleansers.

Some worked for brief periods, and some irritated my sensitive skin and worsened breakouts.

Prologue: Opening up about acne

Acne is much like getting influenza, common cold, or an allergy, it's something you have virtually no control over, and is actually very common. It depends mostly on the skin type you were born with, your genetic history (Yes, one of the most common causes of acne is simply that your parents had it too, passed it down to you), and your environment. Factors like hygiene and your skincare routine diet can trigger acne, but only if you're already likely to get it.

And yet, despite this, the general perception is the reverse. People blessed with clear skin are not more conscious of their habits or stricter in their regimens. Since the world practically runs on appearances, people tend to get very funny about acne (and other skin disorders), generally being sympathetic, expressing regret, or eager to offer their counsel. Now, desperate as I was, I tried out quite a few of these remedies, to little avail.

Over the years, while I was dealing with breakouts and trying out various treatments with little effect, I'd always end up going down internet rabbit holes, websites that offered their advice on the best ways to deal with acne. Yet, almost none of them had a verified, complete, concise guide. That's what this book is. Acne is one of the most complicated skin conditions, a vast field whose exact machinations are still unknown to researchers and specialists. Yet, this book is meant only to help you figure out what works best for your skin and offer companionship as you go through it. Since I would hate to be one of the people providing uncorroborated advice, Dr. Parul Khot has kindly offered to share her expertise, review the medical science behind it all, and recommend some tips.

Eeshta Bhatt

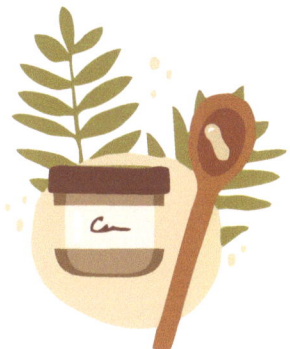

Prologue: Opening up about acne

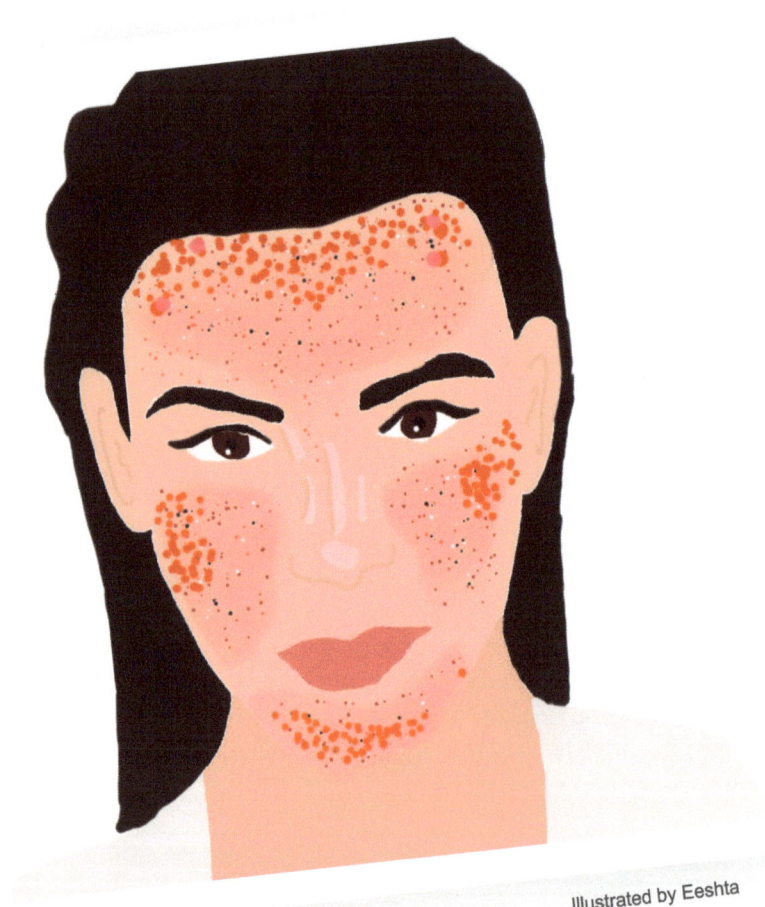

Illustrated by Eeshta

The Basics

Chapter 1

Chapter 1

The Basics

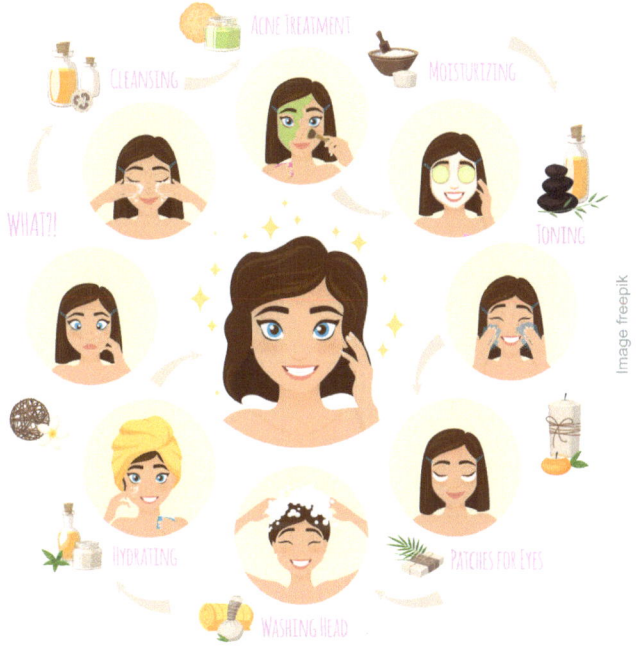

Acne is a multifactorial disease of the sebaceous glands prevalent in teenagers and middle age (adult). It is characterized by the development of several bumps and spots, including blackheads, whiteheads, papules, pustules, nodules, cysts.

But, you're more likely to hear the words pimples, acne, zits, or boils thrown around in various combinations.

Terminology Check: These are all different

- Acne is an umbrella term for a disease that results in the appearance of spots.
- A pimple or a zit is a single inflamed, infected bump.
- A lesion is a dermatological term for an abnormality or mark on the skin; spots are lesions. Acne types like blackheads, whiteheads that we'll cover later on, are also lesions.

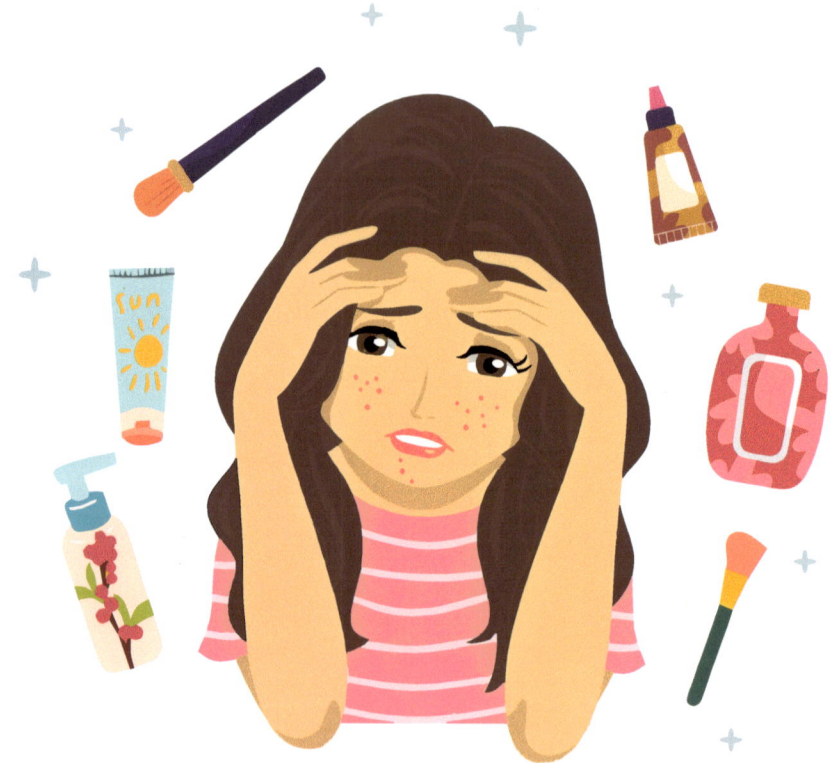

Why is acne interlinked with puberty and your teenage years?

During puberty, both boys and girls experience a hormone surge; the body works overtime, releasing male and female hormones. Androgens, of which testosterone is the principal hormone in men, maintain and are responsible for developing male sex hormones and muscles, bone strength in girls. Too much of it, as can sometimes happen, leads to acne.

Chapter 1: The Basics

1.1 Let's talk numbers

Statistics can be unreliable since they will generally be compiled from dermatology clinics or survey data from a specific population. Hence, I like to think that the data is underrepresented and not an exact reflection of the actual.

Yet, for me, the numbers are reassuring,

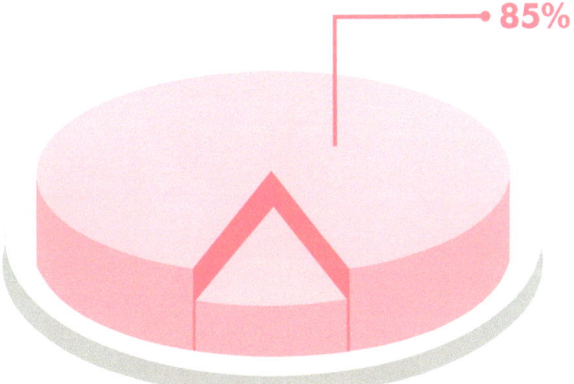

85%

- About 85% of people between the ages of 12-25 have acne.

- Teenage acne is much more frequent than adult acne.

- Among adolescents, most girls will experience acne at the ages of 14-17; boys commonly experience it a little later, from 16-19. There are exceptions, of course.

- 12-20% of adults also struggle with acne, although women are more likely to break out than men due to hormonal changes.

It is easy to conclude that an awful ton of people suffer from acne at least some point in their life. You're far from alone.

Chapter 1: The Basics

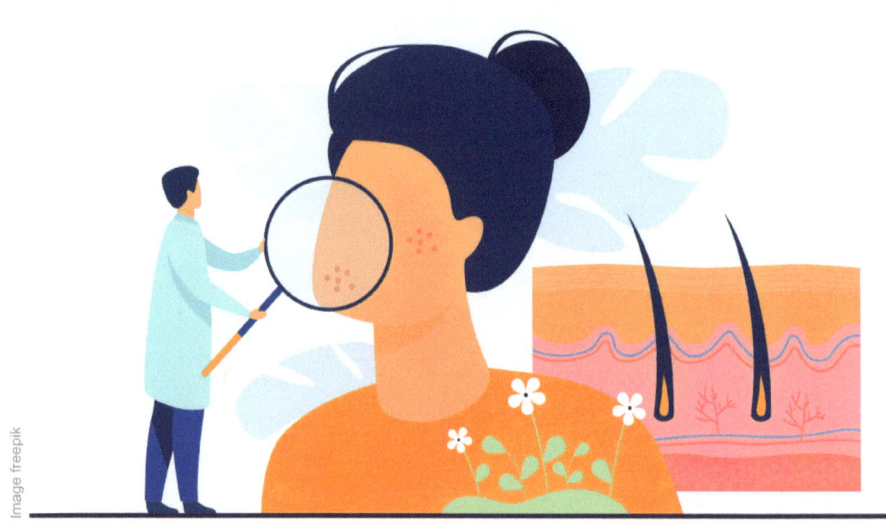

Image freepik

Most skin conditions, mind you, not all, result from hormonal changes in the body. Hormones are chemical messengers circulated in the blood to act on targeted body tissues. Skin changes are often related to variations in the level of sex hormones – testosterone, estrogen, and progesterone. Although the causes for the fluctuations in hormone levels will differ depending on several factors (age, genetics, environment), the scientific reactions taking place under your skin, resulting in acne development, will always be the same.

Chapter 1: The Basics

1.2 A Beginner's Guide to the Science behind the development of Acne

Like most systems in the body, a systematic chain of steps must occur for acne to develop:

- At puberty, but it might also happen otherwise: there are large amounts of circulating hormones called androgens.

- Sebaceous glands are sensitive to it, enlargement of glands, and excess secretion of sebum = seborrhea (Sebum keeps your skin from flaking and drying out).

- Glands are attached to hair follicles. Excess cell duplication at gland opening = hyperkeratinisation.

- Sebum and cells band together, blocking the follicle = Plug formation.

- Small white or black bumps (blackheads and whiteheads) appear, called comedones: mild variety of acne.

- This attracts acne bacteria (Propionibacterium acnes) for whom it is the ideal breeding ground.

- It is typically benign, preferring to live on your skin. However, when exposed to sebum rich environments, it invades plugged follicles (comedones) and rapidly reproduces, feeding on sebum.

- Leads to the formation of papules and pustules = moderate grade of acne.

- Infection and inflammation deepens affecting multiple adjacent glands, nodules form = severe grade.

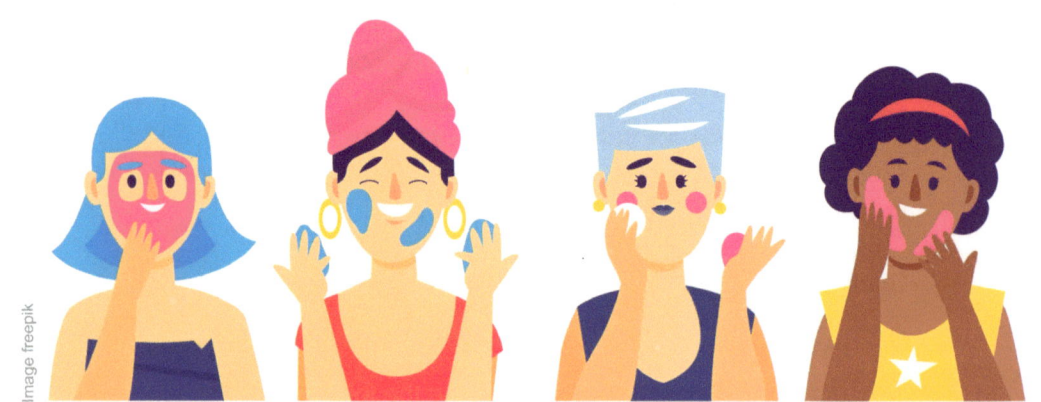

Image freepik

Acne Mapping: How it can help improve your skin?

Your skin is not only the largest organ, but it's the only one that gives you specific visual cues. Although scientists have not been able to crack the acne code, they have figured out an association between inner health and the locations at which acne erupts. This practice was developed 3000 years ago by the Chinese. Called 'mien shiang' (face reading), it considers the face as a map with each section connecting to different organs.

Chapter 1: The Basics

1.3

Getting to know your acne

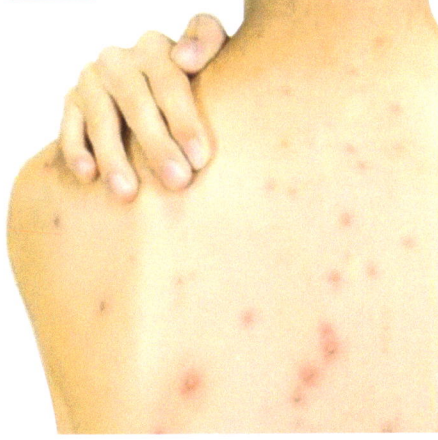

Acne can occur anywhere on the skin having hair follicles, which is well everywhere - although that's depressing. There are two broad classifications, and not everyone develops it everywhere.

There are specific regions where you are more likely to get it, depending on your skin type, genetic history, lifestyle, habits, and other causes that haven't been figured out yet. It's a complicated disorder; however, you can keep track of it all to help you deal with it better.

Body Acne

When you have overactive sebaceous glands, it is not only limited to the ones on your face but glands throughout the skin. Hence, the onset of facial acne is usually marked by bumps on other parts of the body. Some of the most common areas are:

- Arms and shoulders
- Back
- Chest
- Neck
- Torso
- Buttocks

Facial Acne

- Along the hairline
- Temples
- Eyebrows
- Cheeks
- Nose
- Around the mouth/ Upper lip
- Chin
- Jawline
- Forehead

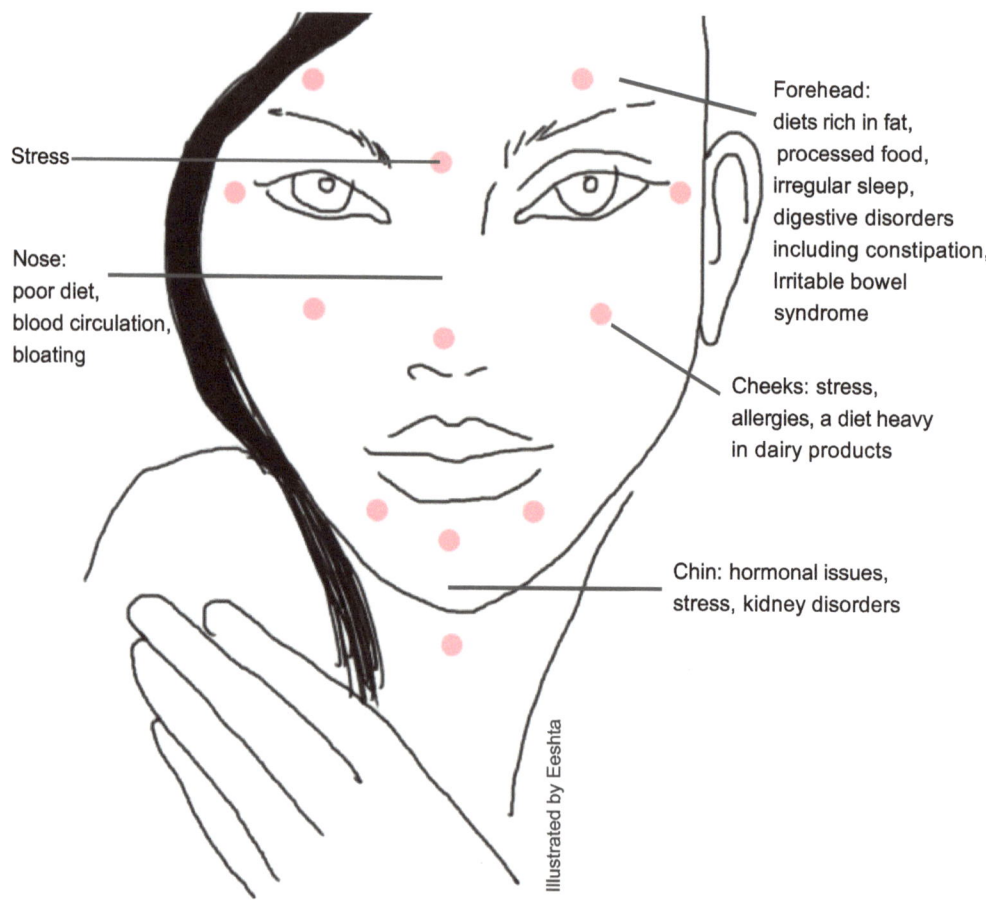

Forehead:
diets rich in fat,
processed food,
irregular sleep,
digestive disorders
including constipation,
Irritable bowel
syndrome

Stress

Nose:
poor diet,
blood circulation,
bloating

Cheeks: stress,
allergies, a diet heavy
in dairy products

Chin: hormonal issues,
stress, kidney disorders

Illustrated by Eeshta

Your body is a complex structure, and it'll let you

know when something isn't quite right.

Acne can be an indicator of conditions associated

with various organ systems.

Chapter 1: The Basics

1.4 Let's get up close and personal with it

Although acne can feel pretty random, suddenly developing on random locations on your face, the specific areas at which acne develops on the face can be indicative of the underlying causes: which can be lifestyle reasons: makeup, cosmetics, habits, or signs that individual organ systems might be malfunctioning. Track the pattern of your outbursts to see your trouble areas and what they may be symptoms of.

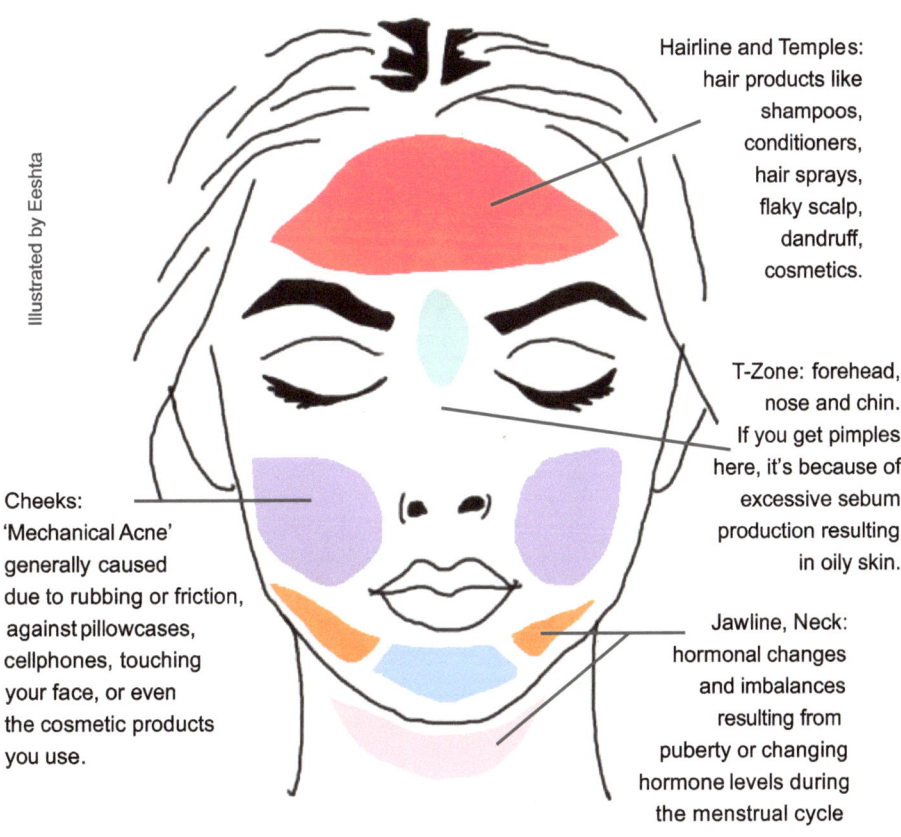

Illustrated by Eeshta

Hairline and Temples: hair products like shampoos, conditioners, hair sprays, flaky scalp, dandruff, cosmetics.

T-Zone: forehead, nose and chin. If you get pimples here, it's because of excessive sebum production resulting in oily skin.

Cheeks: 'Mechanical Acne' generally caused due to rubbing or friction, against pillowcases, cellphones, touching your face, or even the cosmetic products you use.

Jawline, Neck: hormonal changes and imbalances resulting from puberty or changing hormone levels during the menstrual cycle

Chapter 1: The Basics

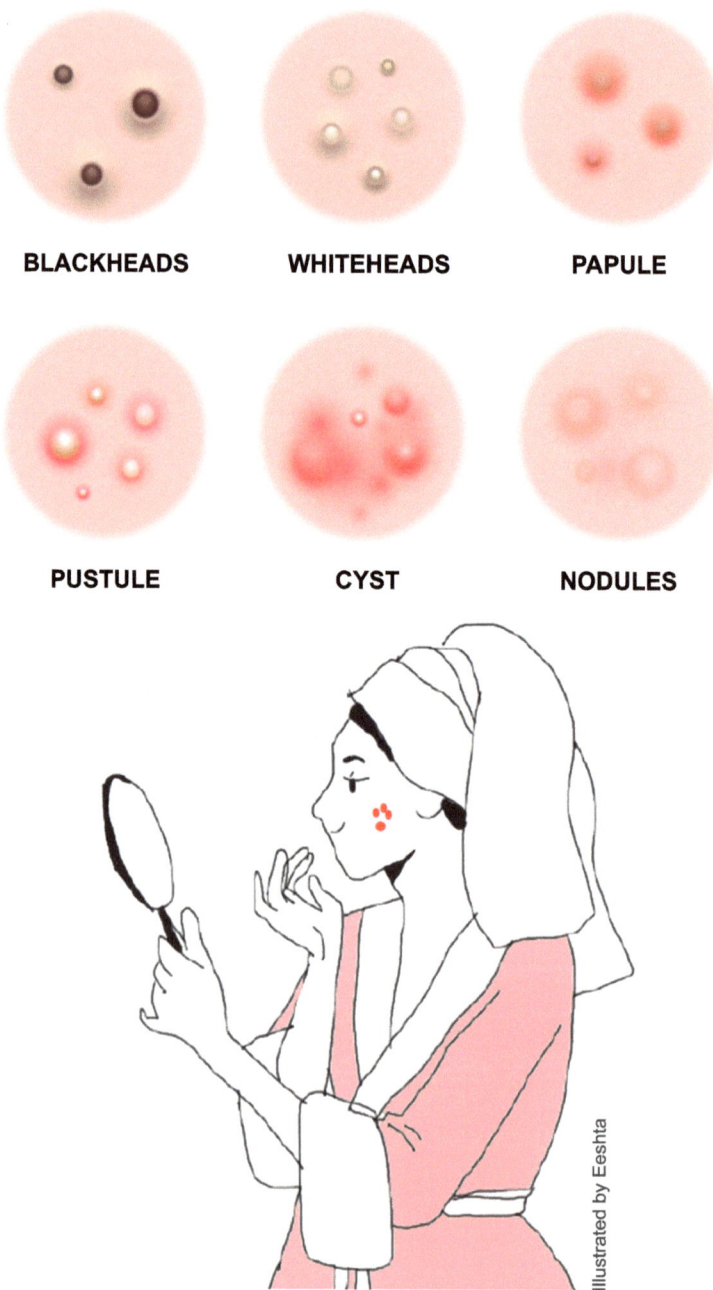

BLACKHEADS   **WHITEHEADS**   **PAPULE**

PUSTULE   **CYST**   **NODULES**

Illustrated by Eeshta

Chapter 1: The Basics

1.5 Classifying Acne

While in most cases, attempting to diagnose yourself is severely warned against, and for a good reason. Googling symptoms rarely ends well, and always comes with a dire warning preparing you for instant health deterioration. This is your chance to go ahead, leap into action and examine yourself.

You need to know what type and form your acne takes. You can either visit your dermatologist or look through the following list, stand at your mirror, and give your acne a long close look. I hated doing this, preferring to forget instead it existed by avoiding every mirror, phone camera placed at proximity.

However, knowing is essential when deciding treatment for over-the-counter remedies or prescription medication.

Non-inflammatory acne: Usually called comedonal acne are characterized by the development of comedones (blackheads and whiteheads). Comedogenesis is a medical term used for the development of blackheads and whiteheads.

Inflammatory acne: Marked by the appearance of papules, pustules, macules, and nodules,cysts.

Blackheads: Black or yellowish, tiny bumps. They're not filled with dirt but are colored because of the lining of the hair follicle.

Whiteheads: Similar to blackheads, but firmer, won't empty when prodded, squeezed.

Papules: Small, firm red bumps, commonly referred to as pimples or zits; are made up of inflammatory blood cells, don't contain pus.

Pustules: Papules that have a white tip in the center, caused by a pus build-up.

Nodules: Large, tender lumps that build-up, and are lodged deeply under the skin.

Cysts: most severe, large pus-filled lumps, very similar to boils, can lead to scarring.

Macule: a flat, red, purple, or brown spot that forms from the remnants of papules and pustules. Macules generally develop after an acne lesion is healing or has healed.

Dr. Parul Khot says:

You're rarely going to see just one acne type, and everyone's skin type is unique and is more likely to experience some acne types than others.

You might see a mixture of whiteheads and blackheads, cysts and blackheads, or any combination of the different types.

You'll find a similar pattern of acne lesions on other parts of the body, most commonly the chest and the back.

Assessing the severity of your Acne

Acne is highly specific, and treatment will be conditional on the grade of your acne. The following chart will help you classify your breakouts according to three brackets:

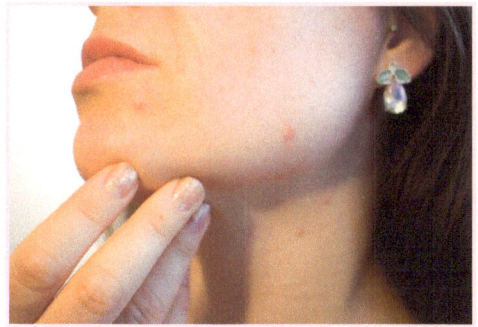

Mild:
Mainly comedones

Moderate Comedones, papules, pustules, macules

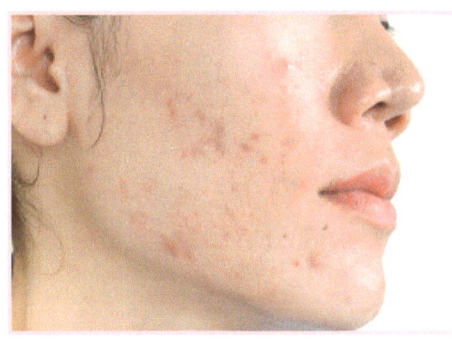

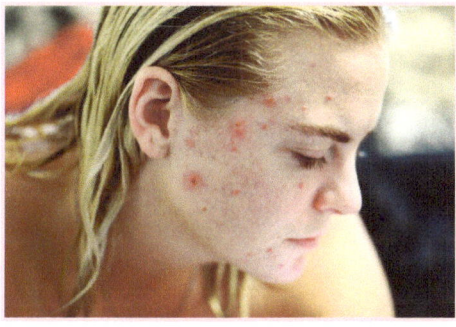

Severe
comedones, papules, pustules, nodules, cysts, macules

There's no definite point at which you should seek advice from a dermatologist. It's a personal experience; some people will require prescription treatment; others may not. However, earlier is always better, so you have time to figure out what works for you.

Chapter 1: The Basics

Is your sleep cycle triggering your breakouts?

At least 7-8 hours of sleep is essential for the optimum functioning of all body systems. During this time, your body delivers fluids to organs and tissues that need replenishing while removing excess fluids from other areas. (This is also why eye bags and dark circles develop). Insufficient sleep causes the stress hormone cortisol to be released, which leads to inflammation, de-stabilizing your immune system and resulting in flare-ups in conditions like acne, psoriasis, and even eczema.

Haircare,Dandruff and Acne

If you experience pimples along your hairline, upper part of your forehead, or your neck, it's almost certainly linked to your haircare routine. Haircare products may contain oil (shampoos, conditioners, serums), which can find its way to your skin, leading to clogged pores and acne. It's crucial to also get rid of residue from these products. Be sure to clean everything your head touched, including pillowcases and sheets, caps, headbands. Dandruff, like acne, is also caused due to oil production. Hence, if you experience one, the other is sure to follow. Further, both have been linked to hormonal fluctuations seen during puberty.

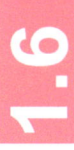

1.6 Causes of acne

Actual reasons that lesions occur can be grouped into two broad headlines: primary causes and triggers that exaggerate pre-existing symptoms:

- Overactive oil glands
- Hormonal changes as in puberty, but breakouts also tend to coincide with the timing of the menstrual cycle
- Diseases relating to the gastrointestinal tract, and digestive system
- Diets having a high glycemic index
- Genetics
- Humidity
- Medications
- Stress either emotional or due to lack of sleep
- Pressure, chafing due to tight clothes, phones, even hair

The hereditary factor

If there is a history of acne in your family, there's a 50% chance of developing it. That's right; you might owe your skin troubles to your genetic history. If both your parents had acne, you have an even greater chance of having it. Why is acne passed down in families?

Just like you inherit your parents' features and skin tone, the genetic information passed down to you in genes contains details that dictate

Certain aspects that affect:
- The functioning of your sebaceous glands like their size, sensitivity, the quantity of sebum they produce
- Pore size, which determines how easily they get clogged
- The ability of your immune system to react to bacteria p. acnes

Common triggers include:
- Local hygiene
- Cosmetic products: sunscreen, moisturizer, makeup, shampoos, conditioners, body wash

Chapter 1: The Basics

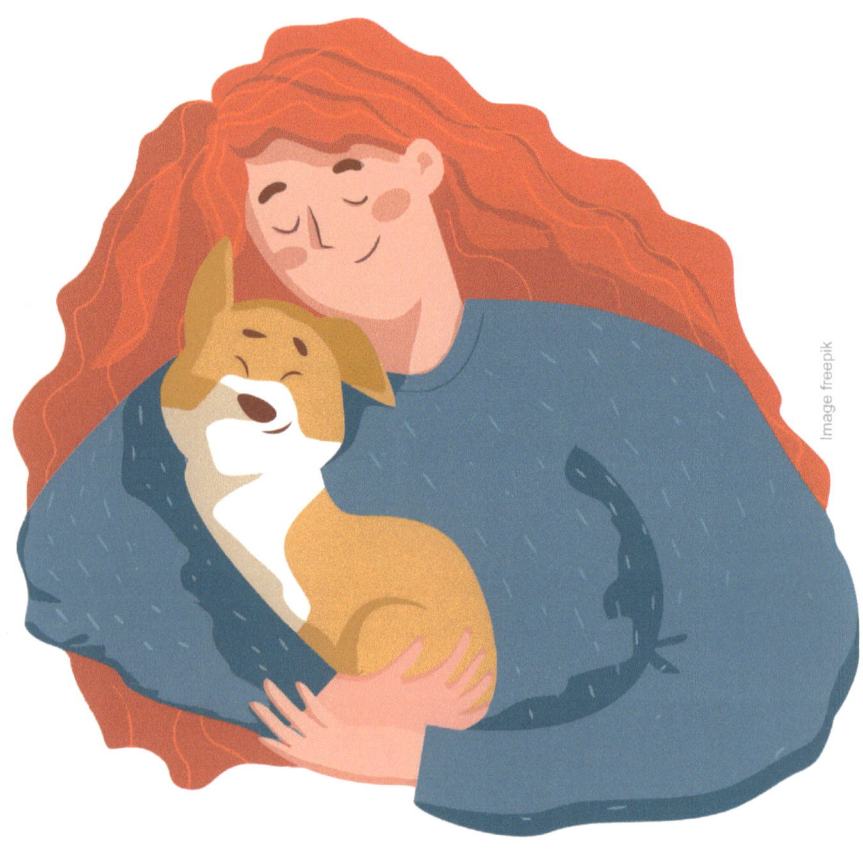

Image freepik

Pet Hair: Can cuddling your furry companion be irritating your skin?

Your pets don't shower every day. The oils, residues, and flea medications that might coat their furs in addition to random dirt and dust they can collect from roaming around can cause breakouts. Further, the ingredients in their shampoo and flea/ tick medications might also contain comedogenic chemicals. Coincidentally your little furry buddy can also get acne for the same reasons as you.

Chapter 1: The Basics

Delving further than skin deep

Chapter 2

Severe Acne

- Nodulocystic acne

- Acne conglobata

- Hyperpigmentation acne

- Acne fulminans

- Keloid and Hypertrophic Scars

Chapter 2

2.1 Severe Acne

▶ Nodulocystic acne

▶ Acne conglobata

▶ Hyperpigmentation acne

▶ Acne fulminans

▶ Keloid and Hypertrophic Scars

Delving further than skin deep

Acne may be a disorder presenting itself on the surface of your skin. Still, it can be linked to drugs taken for other conditions, and issues caused by acne (particularly in its severe form) are rarely skin-deep, resulting in grave consequences for sufferers.

While the previous section outlined some of the primary causes, it's especially important to rule out other potential acne causes linked to specific drugs and medications:

Steroids of two types, (either oral, injected, or inhaled)

- Anabolic steroids that promote musculation - Can lead to the appearance of fungal acne Malassezia folliculitis characterized by itchy superficial papules and pustules will be seen on the chest and back, unlike normal acne vulgaris, all lesions will be similar in size.

- Prescription corticosteroids like prednisone, dexamethasone is given after transplant surgeries.

Anti-psychotic drugs (antidepressants)

Drugs are taken for other diseases, malaria, and tuberculosis:
1. Antituberculosis drugs like rifampicin can cause acne.
2. Anticonvulsants
3. Contraceptives
Acne outbursts are also common during pregnancy and breastfeeding.

2.1 Severe acne

Nodulocystic acne

Affects the face, chest, and back may even develop on the shoulders and behind the ears.
More common in men, women often get in on the lower half of their faces.

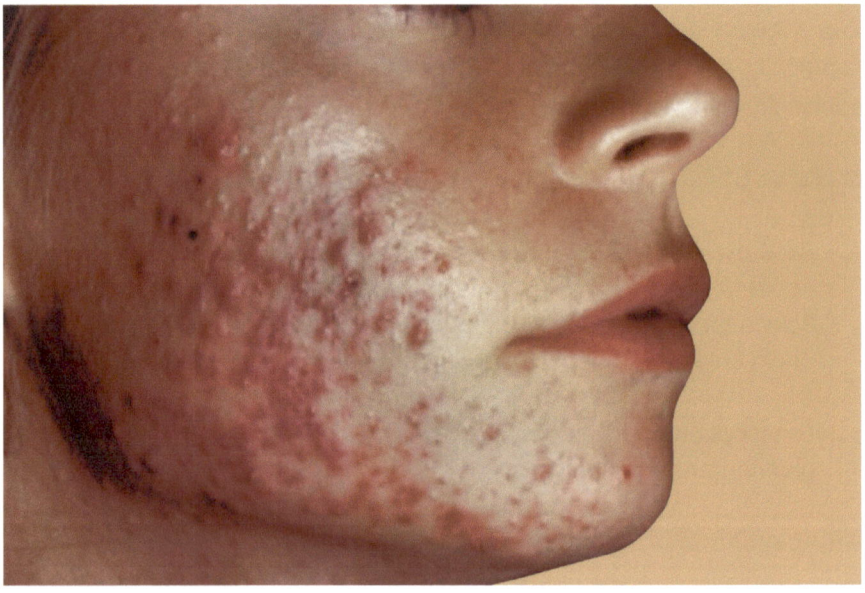

Causes:

- Develops when you have extensive, red, painful breakouts deep in your skin.
- Characterized by multiple inflamed and uninflamed nodules and scars.

Identifying clinical features include:
- Large pus-filled cyst
- Large white bump
- Redness
- Tender or painful to the touch
- Not true cysts as there is no epithelial lining. They are sometimes called pseudocysts.
- If cysts burst, the infection spreads rapidly, causing more breakouts.

Acne conglobata

Acne conglobata is a distinctive form of nodulocystic acne interconnecting abscesses and sinuses (channels under the skin caused due to the combined growth of acne cysts and nodules deep below the skin.

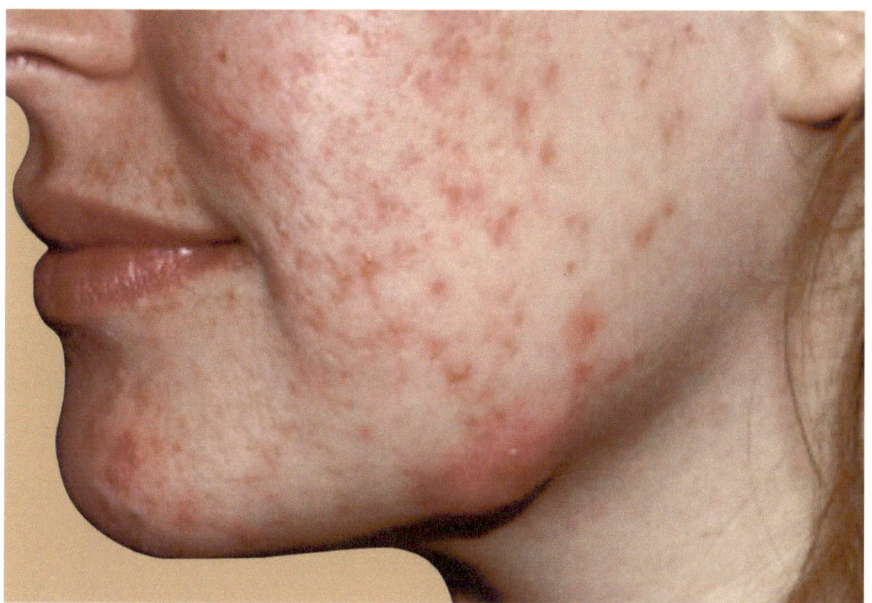

Hyperpigmentation acne

- May occur in all skin types but more frequently in darker skin tones since dark spots result from excess melanin production.

- The color tends to be darker and more intense in dark skin tones and persists for longer durations.

- Certain medications might also blacken post-inflammatory pigmentation. These include antimalarial drugs, anticancer drugs.

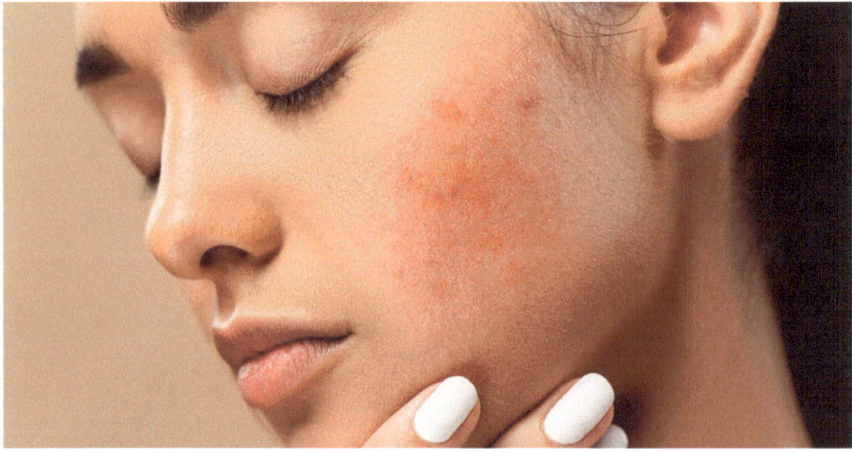

Causes
- Deposition of melanin within keratinocytes (skin cells) results in swelling in the epidermis.
- Melanin synthesis is increased and transferred to surrounding keratinocytes.
- This triggers a cycle of events that causes post-inflammatory hyperpigmentation.

Identifying clinical features include:
- Different from other acne forms because it does not appear as a raised pimple but rather a dark spot or patch on the skin.
- Some hyperpigmentation lesions are deeper since they develop in the dermis, are blue-grey, and can be permanent.

Chapter 2: Delving further than skin deep

Acne fulminans

Acne fulminans is a very severe form of acne conglobata.

Causes
- It is associated with increased levels of androgens, complex autoimmune disease, and a genetic predisposition.
- May also be related to an explosive hypersensitivity reaction to surface bacteria (Cutibacteria acnes).
- Could be triggered by high doses of isotretinoin when treating severe acne and anabolic steroids, although treatment often involves both of these.

Features
- A rare skin disorder presents as an acute, painful, ulcerating, and hemorrhagic clinical form of acne.
- Very sudden onset.
- Patients may experience fevers and widespread joint pain.
- Nodules are painful to touch, ulcerated, hemorrhagic, and sometimes covered with crusts. It differs from acne conglobata in that there are cysts and acutely inflamed lesions, but no polyporous comedones.

Severe acne scars

Again acne is individualistic, so you might be part of the lucky few that have trouble getting rid of acne scars. However, in most cases, very severe forms of acne will leave behind scars in their place.

There are two main types: Keloid and Hypertrophic Scars
- Common types of scarring that occur due to the acne healing process.
- Typically develop on the chest, back, and shoulders, where the skin is thicker, although they can occur around the jawline.
- Incidence is higher in people with darker skin types.
- A keloid scar is larger than the acne lesion that caused it.
  A hypertrophic scar is the same size as the acne lesion that caused it.

Chapter 2: Delving further than skin deep

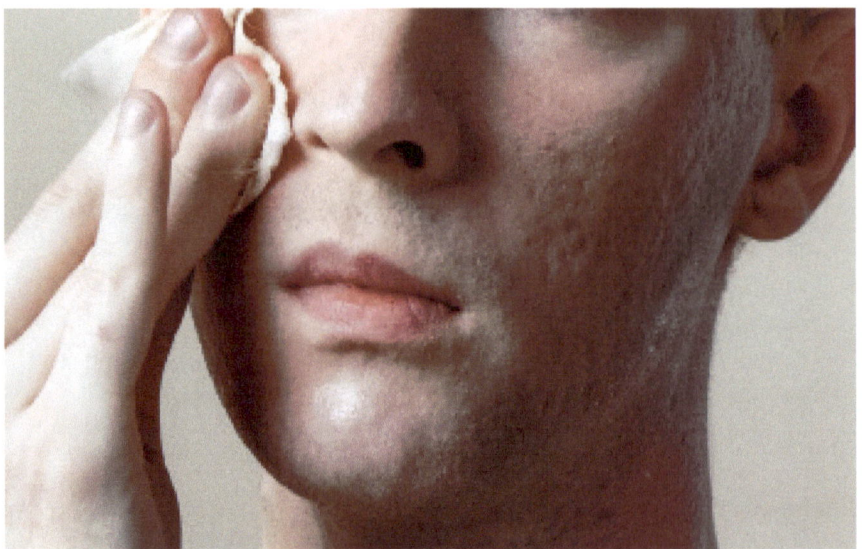

Causes or factors that trigger their formation

Result from the overgrowth of fibrous tissue in the region where the acne lesion had developed.
- Dependent on the ability of the skin to heal.
- Skin types that tend to scar easily are more likely to have keloids and hypertrophic scars.
- Picking or squeezing acne lesions can damage the skin.
- Darker skin types have several genetic factors that significantly increase the likelihood of thickened scars.

Identifying clinical features
- Hard, firm, lumpy scars
- Appear as raised lesions of scar tissue on the skin

Hygiene

Chapter 3

Chapter 3

Hygiene

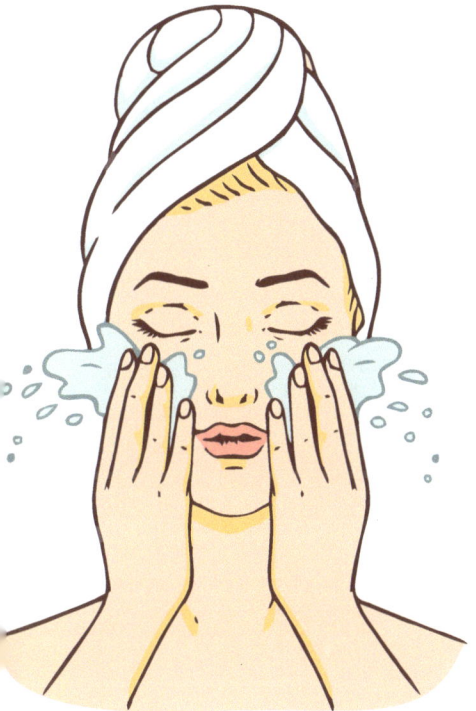

Acne is caused due to excessive oil production, not poor hygiene. When I was younger, I used this as an argument to avoid washing my face multiple times a day when at school or against changing pillow covers.

However, I failed to understand that hygiene can trigger acne, and although acne is very rarely preventable, proper skin care is essential for its management and treatment.

Excess accumulation of oil on the skin attracts dirt and other particles, leading to infection. Even something as small as not having your hair tied back and changing your napkins and pillowcases can result in breakouts.

General Advice

Before we get into the specifics, here's a specially compiled list of Do's and Don't's arranged by Dr. Parul Khot. Leaf through them at your leisure, general advice when dealing with acne-prone skin, and identify flaws in your skincare routines.

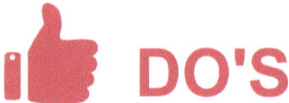 # DO'S

- Facial skin that is prone to pimples must be kept clean.
- Wash your face twice a day with lukewarm water (generally morning and night).
- Wash your hair regularly and tie your hair back. Loose hair on your skin can agitate it, leading to acne.
- Unclean hair and dandruff result in breakouts.
- Shower immediately after physical activity.
- If you wear glasses, wash them regularly to prevent oil and sweat from accumulating that leads to clogged pores.
- Change your pillowcases every 2-3 days and wipe down your phone screen to remove dirt and bacteria from touching your face.
- Use cleansers, toners, moisturizers, and sunscreens that suit your skin type. You can do this with the information provided in the next chapter or with help from your dermatologist.

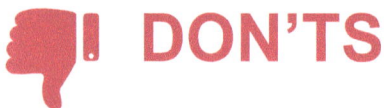 # DON'TS

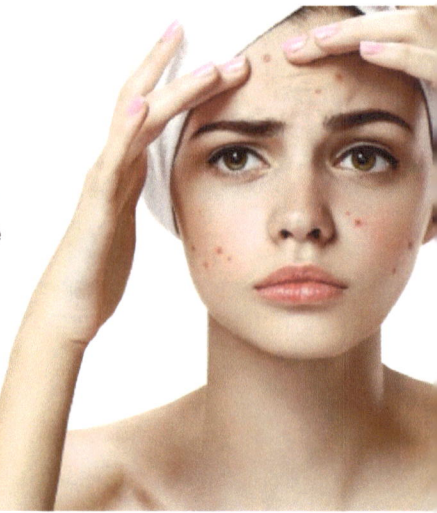

- Do not touch your face except when necessary.
- Avoid squeezing and picking at acne lesions; this will significantly increase the risk of scarring.
- Do not use facial scrubs if you have active acne; this will lead to rashes.
- Avoid over washing your face to prevent dryness and the formation of reddish patches.

3.1 CTMS: The Fearsome Foursome

Cleanser, Moisturizer, Toner, Sunscreen

So skincare routines might seem like they belong in the realm of beauty bloggers, complicated rituals that last for hours into the night, interfering with the urge to just climb into bed, in pyjamas with your phone lined up to a Netflix binge or mindless YouTube video, but they're slightly misjudged.

We're going to focus on four products before concentrating on acne medications in the next section. The skin is classified into four basic categories: oily, dry, combination, and sensitive. You should know which category or categories your skin falls under since this decides which products and chemical will best suit your face.

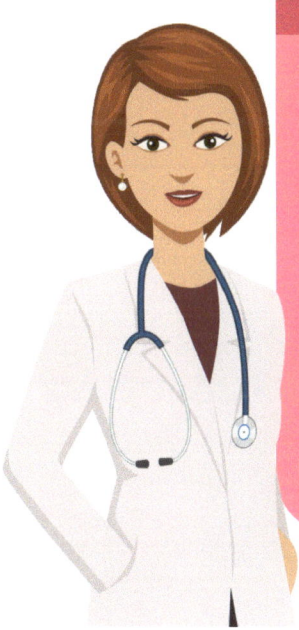

Dr. Parul Khot says:

A simple solution to find out your skin type:

1. Wash your face, dry with a soft clean towel.
2. Wait for 10 minutes.
3. Dab with tissue paper, leave it on for 5 minutes.
4. If the tissue is mainly soggy: you have oily skin.
5. If it's primarily dry: you have dry skin.
6. Combination: when parts are oily and dry.

CLEANSERS

BEST INTERNATIONAL BRANDS

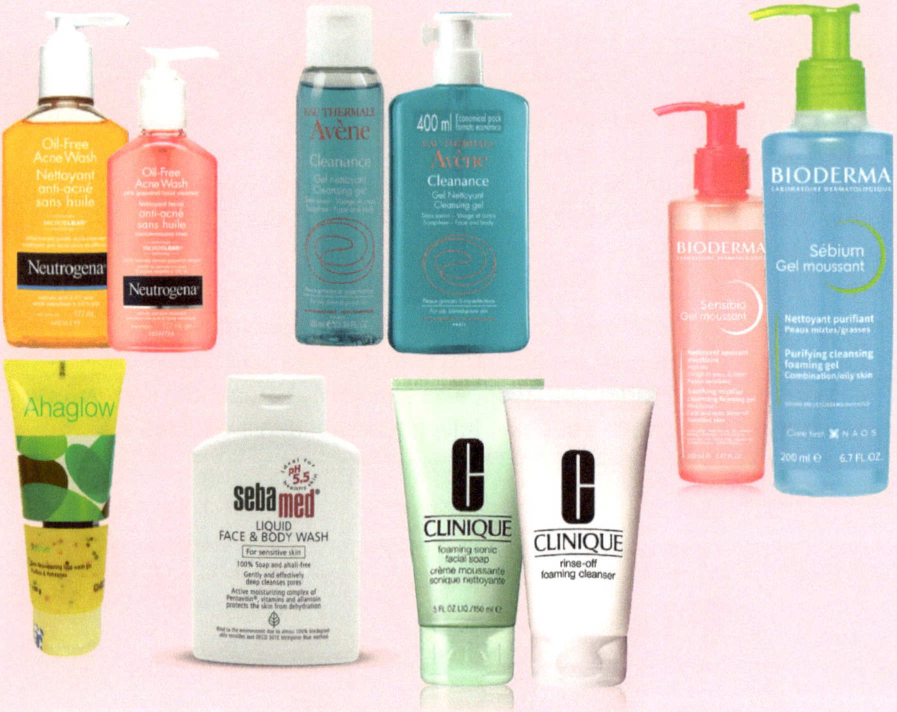

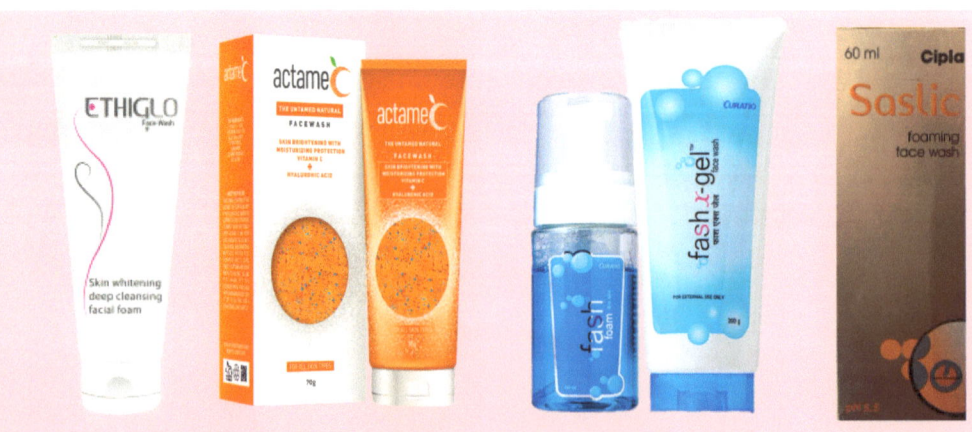

BEST INDIAN BRANDS

Chapter 3: Hygiene

3.2 Cleanser For Acne Prone Skin

A cleanser is just a fancier name for the face wash you need to use. It's incredibly tricky to clean skin that's prone to breakouts and sensitivity without irritating it. Further, a thorough refreshing cleanse is crucial for treating breakouts and minimizing future acne flare-ups

It is always best to experiment. I've gone through a number of cleansers, and still use at least two of them at a time depending on whether my skin is normal, drying, or oily.

Consider the following points before you buy a cleanser:

- It should suit your skin. (but for that you should know your skin type)
- Should be non-comedogenic
- Should not be heavy or oil-based.
- Any oil-based products are a definite no for acne-prone skin.
- Your cleanser should deep cleanse your skin but not over-cleanse it.
- Should not irritate your skin. Avoid products that burn or itch.
- Strictly avoid harsh chemicals that can make breakouts worse by drying and irritating your skin.
- A good cleanser provides you with a 'fresh' feel, leaving your skin soft and clean.

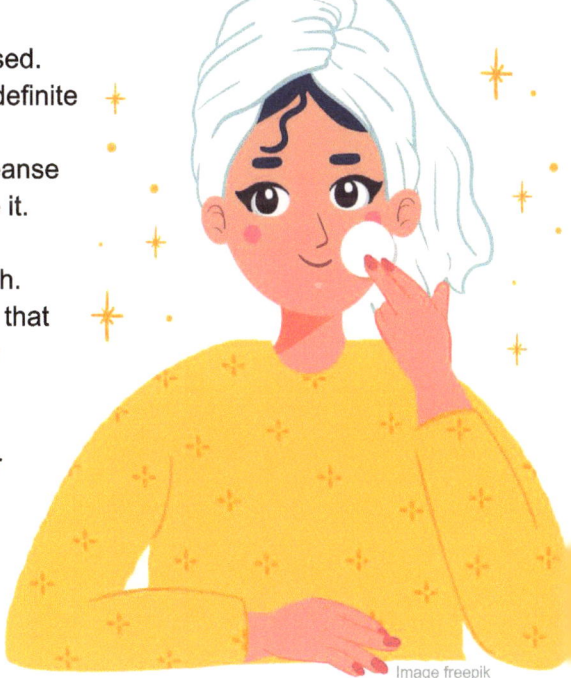

Image freepik

Chapter 3: Hygiene

TEXTURE IS KEY

Using the word 'texture' might seem like we're food connoisseurs reviewing dishes, but cleansers come in different formulations:
There are cleaning foams, gels, moisturizing washes. Water-based and gel-based ones are always better. Go with what feels right for you. Follow your instincts. Unlike other disorders, your skin will always give you prompt feedback, through visual clues. Redness, itchiness after a wash is not a good sign.

Note: Over cleansing/ frequent washing strips your skin of its natural oils, disrupts pH balance.

How can you tell?
Over cleaned skin feels tight and dry i.e, if you find it difficult to move your mouth and stretch your facial skin.

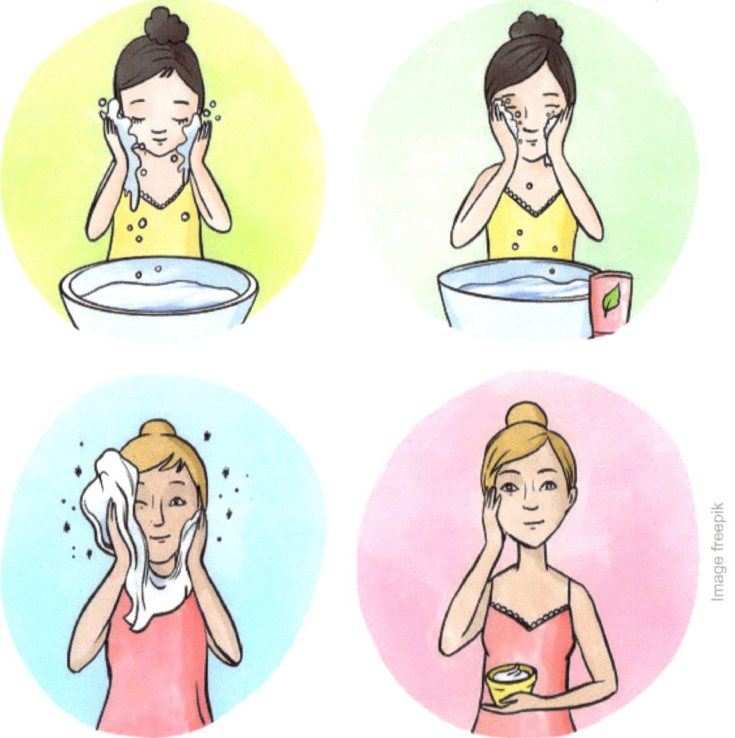

Image freepik

Chapter 3: Hygiene

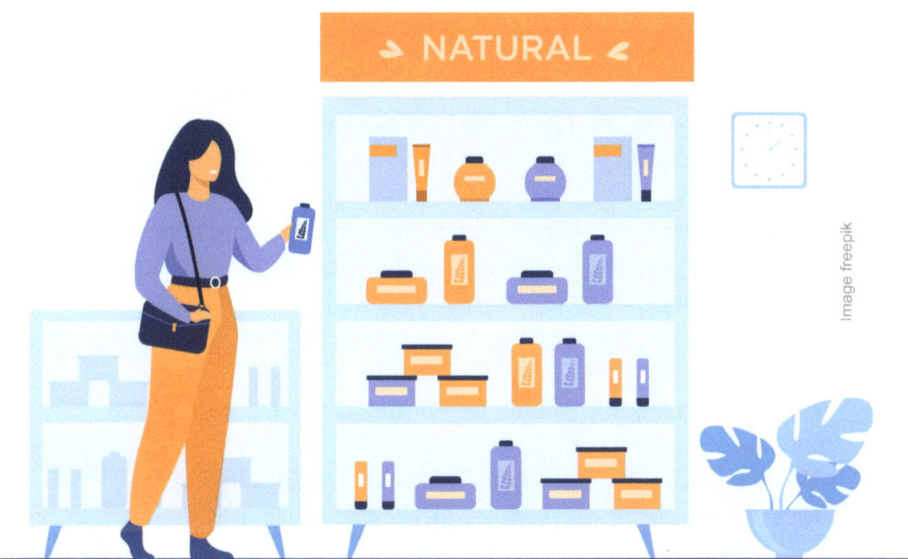

Image freepik

Let's Shop

I used to go by brands that I found suited me, or yes, sometimes color and smell. Not a very sound strategy, I know. The best is to turn the product over and have a look at the ingredients label.

Focus on finding the following compounds:
Fruit acids like
- Salicylic Acid (BHA-beta hydroxy acid)
- Glycolic Acid (AHA-alpha hydroxy acids)
- Benzoyl Peroxide
- Niacinamide

Why? Cleansers with these ingredients
- Penetrate pores
- Unclog them
- Reduce the size of comedones
- Slow the formation of new ones

Chapter 3: Hygiene

Ingredient Spotlight

What's so great about them?
Let's have a quick look at the scientific and chemical nature of these ingredients that make them miracle workers: Formulations containing salicylic acid and benzoyl peroxide are usually harsher and have a stronger effect on the skin, making them best suited for oily skin.

Topical Salicylic acid: A fruit acid, soluble in oil, and is able to break an oily film and go deep into glands, removing trapped dirt, hair, and excess sebum trapped in pores, ensuring a deep cleanse.

Beta-hydroxy acid: Fat or oil-soluble
- Dissolves in fat, and sebum penetrates deep into sebaceous
- glands.
- Unclogs pores at their depth and reduces inflammation.
  Most formulations will have up to 1-2% salicylic acid.

Glycolic Acid: Belongs to a class of fruit acids that are soluble in water, very effective at removing dirt and particles from the surface of your skin.

Alpha hydroxy acids: Water-soluble
- Derived from sugarcane
- Remove excess oil
- Is a natural exfoliant, hence removes dead skin cells and impurities from the surface of the skin.
- Typical concentration: 2-5%

Benzoyl Peroxide: Antibacterial compound, which kills acne bacteria, P. acnes.
- Used to treat mild to moderate acne
- Antibacterial exfoliant
- Works like an antiseptic attack acne bacterium and unclogs pores by removing dead skin cells.

- Typical concentrations: 2.5-10% for both prescription and over the counter treatment
- Generally, face washes will be 2.5-5%

Niacinamide: A form of Vitamin B3 soothes your skin while cleaning it, reducing inflammation, and redness.
- Vitamin B3 derivative
- It is a calming agent.
- Reduces inflammation and size of acne lesions
- It has a protective effect on the skin.
- Also reduces marks and scars left behind by lesions
- If you have dry/sensitive skin, products containing niacinamide are a must buy.

Cleansing FAQ's

How do you use a cleanser to achieve the best effect?

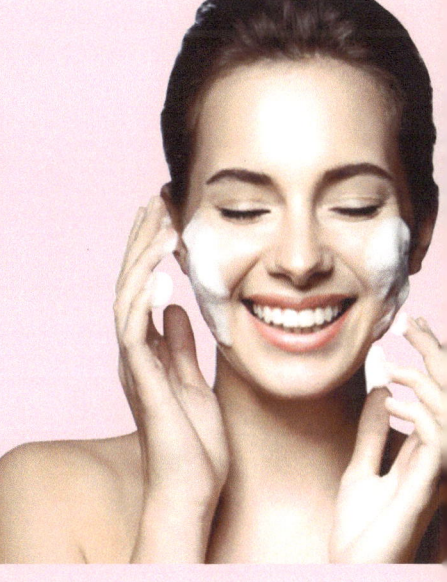

- Wet your face with lukewarm water.
- Always use your fingertips only to gently massage cleanser onto your face.
- Take your time; up to a minute is the recommended time for the product to cleanse the face properly
- Do not scrub; this will irritate your skin.
- Rinse with lukewarm water and pat dry with a fresh, soft, clean towel.

I mistakenly believed that scrubbing with a towel produced the best effects. However, scrubbing vigorously only smoothens the surface of your skin, doing nothing for the infection underneath and aggravating your skin in the process.

Chapter 3: Hygiene

TONERS

BEST INTERNATIONAL BRANDS

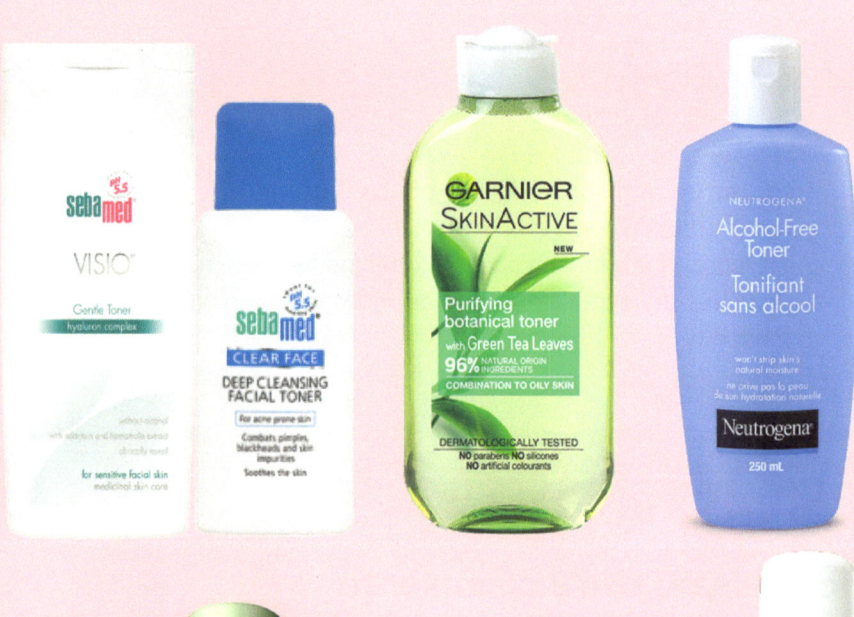

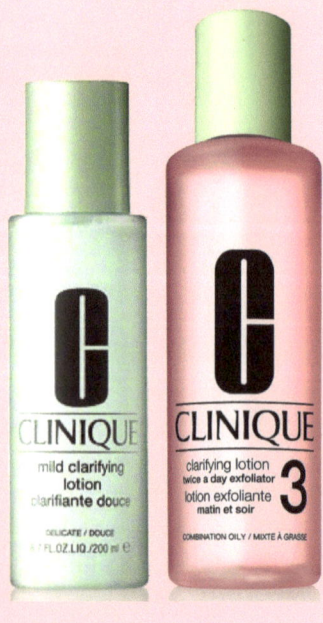

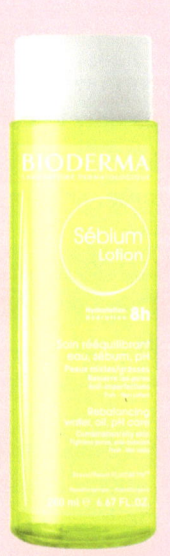

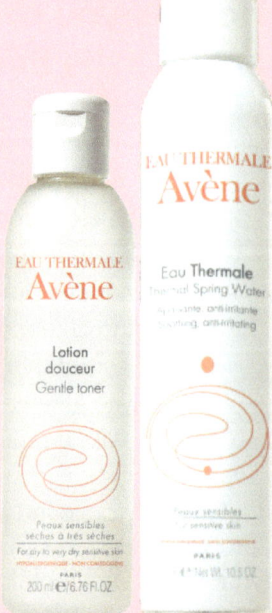

Chapter 3: Hygiene

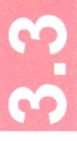

3.3 Toner

Toners can generally be foregone except when applying makeup. Applying toner and moisturizer before you start applying other products including primers, foundation ensures the make-up does not penetrate deep into your skin and stays on the surface. We'll go over this in later sections.

- A toner is hugely beneficial for 'oily' acne-prone skin.
- It is a must-have skincare product if you use heavy makeup skin products.
- Especially important when dealing with adult acne, often caused by heavy makeup worn daily in a professional environment.

TONER FAQ's

How and when should you apply toner?

Generally, toner is applied twice a day. However, if your skin begins to feel dry or irritated, you can limit to once a day, in the morning before you apply your makeup or even every other day.
Pour a small amount of toner onto a cotton ball, dab cotton ball gently over your face.

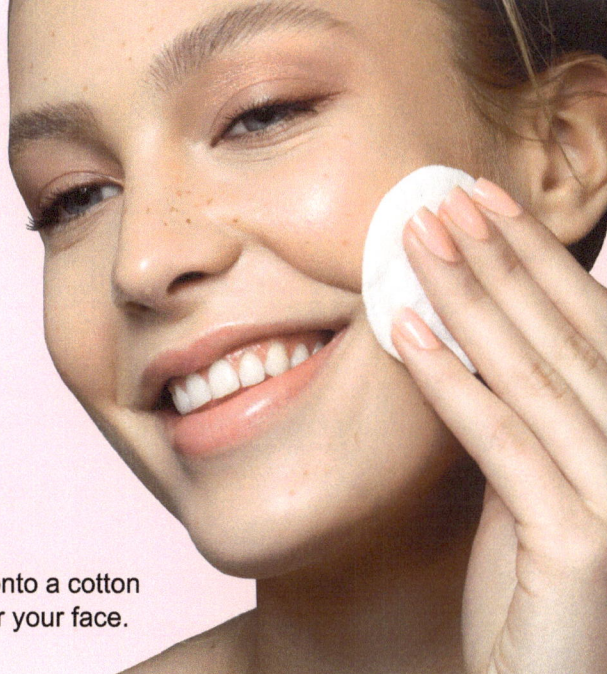

Chapter 3: Hygiene

Key ingredients to look out for:

- Natural fruit acids like salicylic acid, glycolic acid, and lactic acid
  Why?: Remove excess oil, clears skin, freshens complexion without stripping the skin of its natural oils.
- Natural ingredients like cucumber, tea tree, rose water, green tea
- Water-based, freshening, mild, and cleansing without irritating your skin, while forming a protective barrier to prevent makeup from seeping into your skin and aggravating your acne.
- Your toner must be alcohol-free.
- Alcohols (not spirits, drinking kind, or rubbing alcohol) are added to products for two purposes as solvents (ethyl alcohol) that increase water solubility but can be dehydrating and moisturizing fatty alcohols (stearyl, cetyl) that tend to irritate your skin and clog pores.

Watch Out! Plant-Based Is Not Always Good

A reasonable conclusion to make would be to go for all-natural organic products, with no added chemicals. Not always true. Moisturizing alcohols are often derived from vegetable sources. Also, plant oils are notoriously comedogenic, so steer clear of any products containing them.

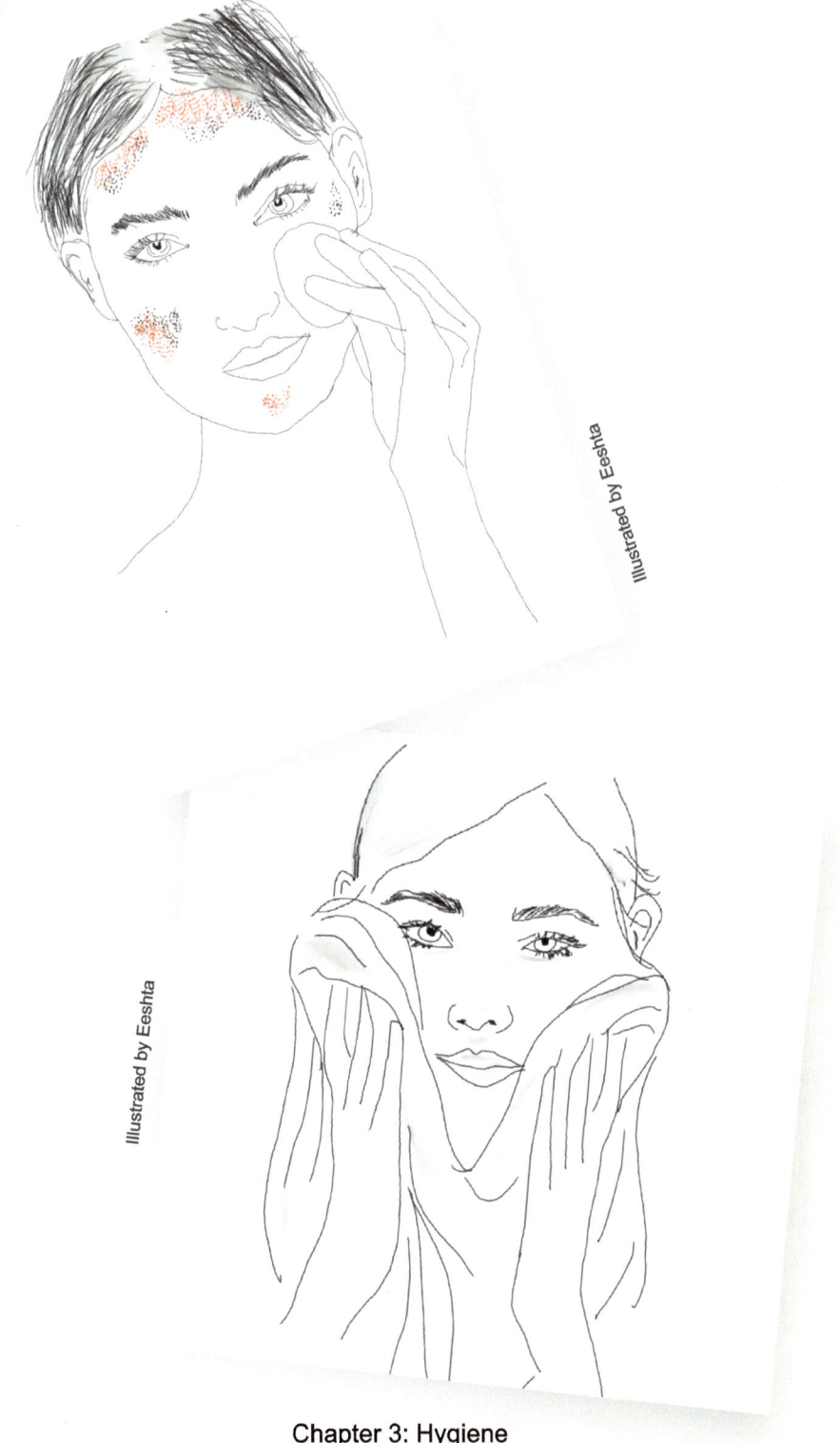

Illustrated by Eeshta

Illustrated by Eeshta

Chapter 3: Hygiene

MOISTURIZERS

BEST INTERNATIONAL BRANDS

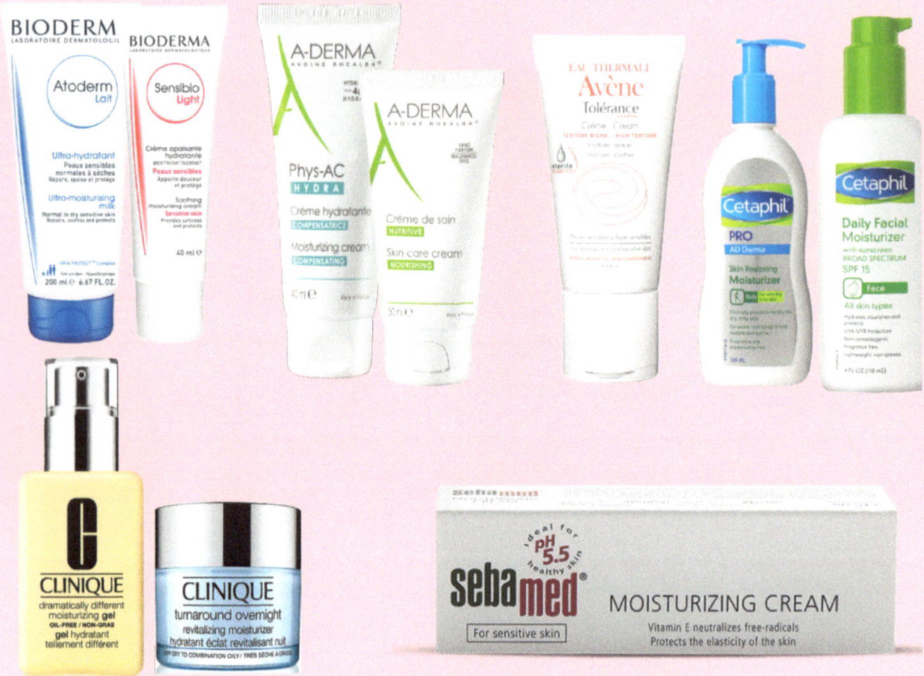

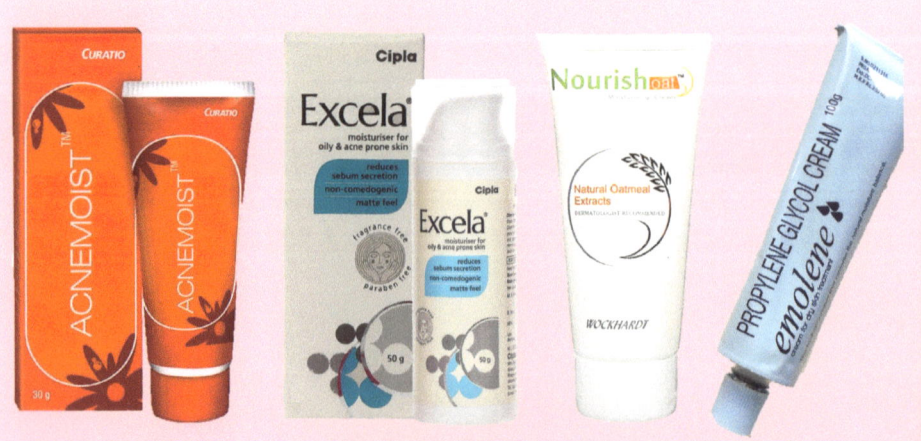

BEST INDIAN BRANDS

Chapter 3: Hygiene

3.4 Moisturizers

It might seem counter-intuitive to use a moisturizer for oily acne-prone skin. I certainly never used one until this year for fear that it would be oily, itchy and aggravate my skin. However, what follows is a repeating cycle of oily skin, followed by dry, flaky skin due to ointments, and drugs.

Contrary to what you might think, dry skin flaking off will only lead to itchiness, and more breakouts, rather than a fresh smooth layer of skin appearing in its place.

Here's why a moisturizer must be a part of your skincare routine:
- Hydration of your skin is essential to repair and nourish damaged acne skin.
- Acne medications, used systematically, can lead to dryness that worsens breakouts. Moisturizers counter this.
- Moisturizers calm the skin, reducing inflammation, and making sure it doesn't penetrate deeper layers.

Characteristics of a good moisturizer:
- Water-based
- Texture matters! Avoid cream or ointment-based moisturizers.
- Look for light formulations (lotions) and gel-based products.
- Matte Finish: should leave your skin feeling soft without being greasy.
- Noncomedogenic: doesn't clog pores
- Reduces sebum secretion

Key Ingredients to look out for:
Niacinamide, Glycerine, Zinc, Allantoin, Ceramides
- These ingredients help recreate the skin's natural moisture by supporting the water and lipid balance in the epidermis.
- Reduce sebum production by inhibiting the multiplication of sebum-producing cells.

Ingredient Spotlight

Allantoin: Plant-based compound, that hydrates your skin, removes dead skin cells, and reduces redness.
- Non-toxic compound found in plants like chamomile, wheat sprouts, comfrey (a purple flowery herb), sugar beet
- A moisturizing agent that provides hydration
- Exfoliant
- Soothing and wound healing properties
- Proliferates cells, reducing dullness
- Synthesizes collagen that holds skin together, anti-ageing properties

Note: Must not be used with fruit acids (AHA's and BHA's)

Ceramides: A type of fat, naturally found in the skin, that holds it together, protecting it against external elements.
- Fats (lipids) concentrated in the uppermost layers of the skin
- Hold the skin together by forming a barrier that limits moisture loss, protects against other environmental threats: pollution, sun
- Sun damage can deplete them
- Products containing ceramides will restore skin's barrier, have a hydrating effect on your skin

Note: Lose their effectiveness when exposed to sunlight and air

Hyaluronic Acid and Glycerin
Both HA and Glycerin are humectants, which means they can draw water from the environment into the skin to create long-lasting hydration. Molecules of HA can also hold large quantities of water, up to several times their weight, thereby ensuring deep hydration and giving your skin a plumper, smoother feel.

Tea Tree
It has anti-inflammatory and antimicrobial properties and can calm redness, swelling, and inflammation. It may even help to prevent and reduce **acne** scars.

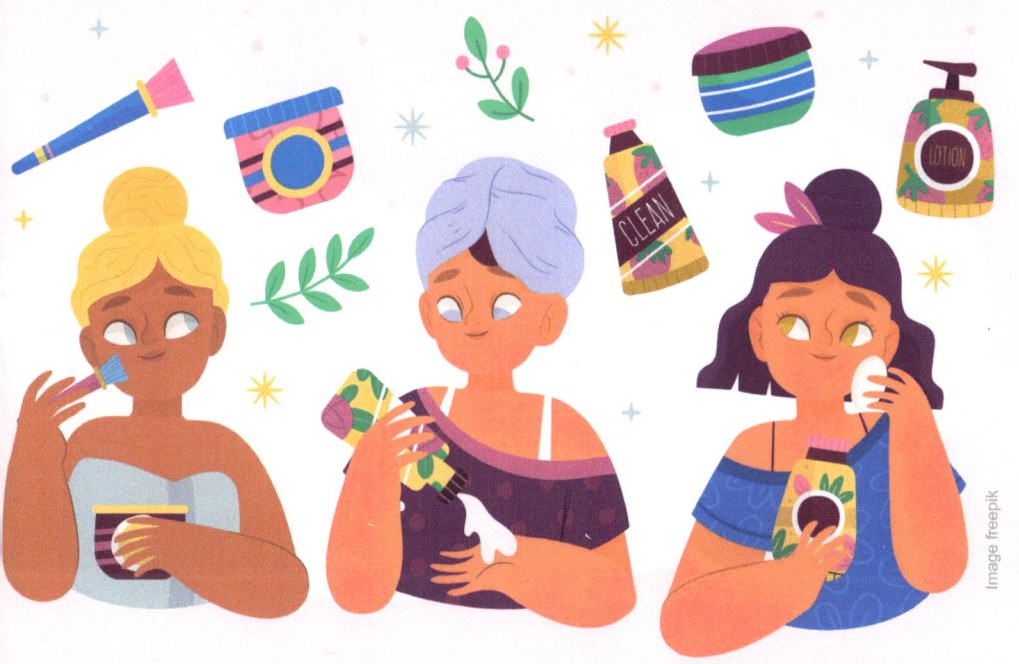

Image freepik

Skin Stories: Pimple Popping

An extremely popular iPad app when I was growing up was 'Pimple Popper.' The interface displayed a character with a terrible flare-up of pustules. The player would have to squeeze the pus out of it; the graphics were nasty but not severe enough to make you cringe. The pimples would leave no marks in their place, and clear shining skin would prevail. Unfortunately, it doesn't quite work that way in real life as much as I, and I'm sure countless others wished it did.

As a general rule, you should never attempt to burst a pimple. You could damage your skin barrier, risking scarring. Far from being a quick fix, it can also delay your skin's natural healing process. That being said, if you cannot resist the urge, only attempt to do so for blackheads and whiteheads. Never for a nodule or a cyst. After applying an over-the-counter acne cream, and washing your hands thoroughly, apply pressure to both sides of the clogged pore to extract the plug.

Chapter 3: Hygiene

SUNSCREEN

BEST INTERNATIONAL BRANDS

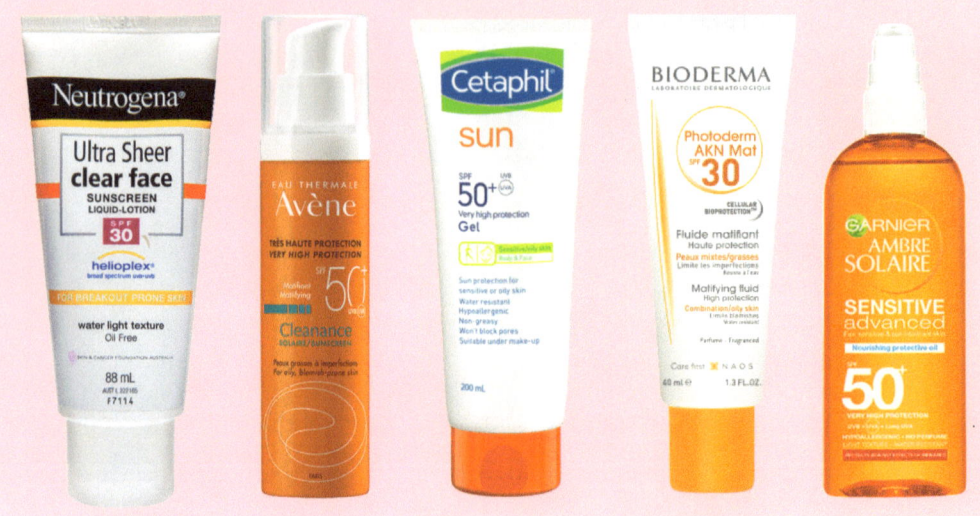

BEST INDIAN BRANDS

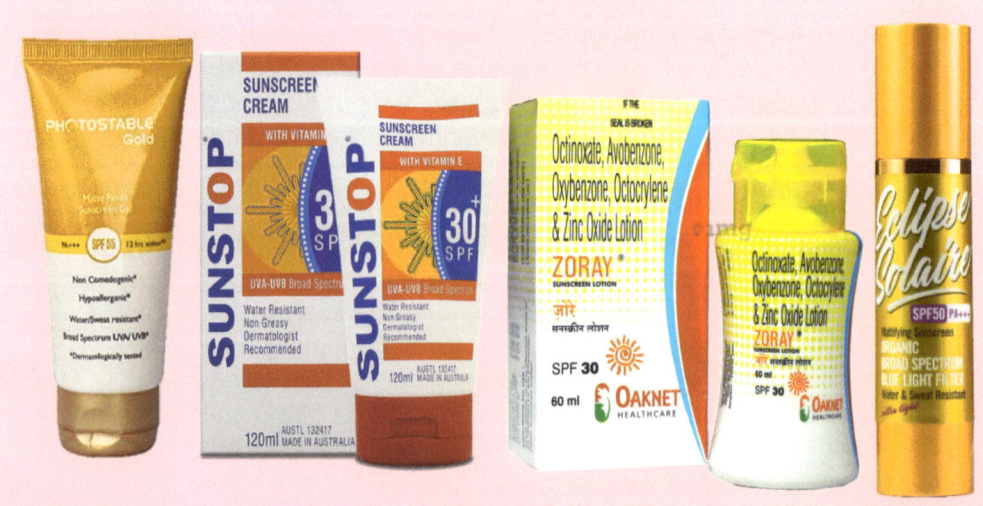

Chapter 3: Hygiene

3.5 Sunscreen

Why you need sunscreen?

- Oily skin is inflamed skin sensitive to external bacteria since the skin's barrier is broken.
- Sunscreens protect your skin from external pollutants and environmental UV rays.

Further, acne medications like Retinol, Benzoyl Peroxide, Glycolic Acid, and Isotroin, among others, are photosensitive, demand strict protection against the sun. For sensitive skin, sunscreen can be irritating. I would always put it on and then scrub it off within minutes, due to an itchy, uncomfortable sensation that I knew was signaling a breakout.

However, this is simply a matter of pros and cons. Let's draw up a list. In the long run, you're better off with it than without-a bit of a bummer.

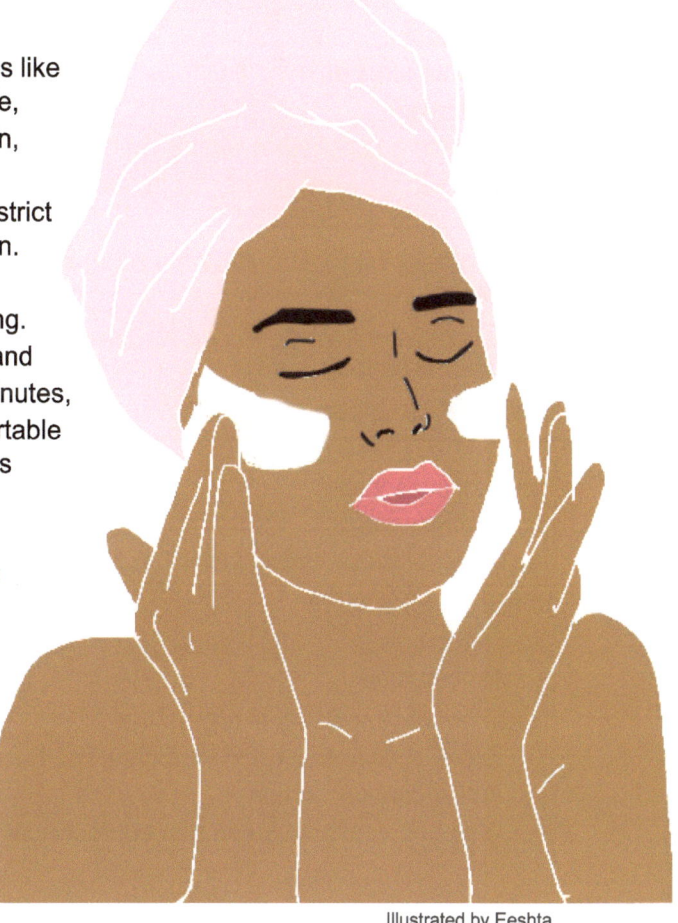

Illustrated by Eeshta

Chapter 3: Hygiene

Characteristics of a good sunscreen

- Lightweight
- Water-based (aqua-based)
- Gel-based
- Water-resistant
- Matte finish (silicone base)
- SPF: 15-30

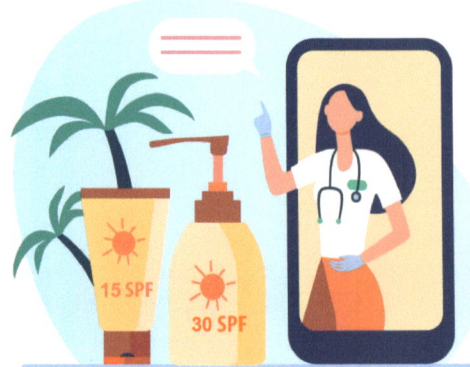

Remember, all your products should bear the label of non-comedogenic.

How do you use it? Application Tips

- Use the 13-dot technique to apply your sunscreen to your face and neck.
- This ensures an even finish, so your skin is evenly covered and protected.
- It has to be applied at least 20 minutes before going out in the sun
- The skin may feel greasy for the first five minutes, but give it some time to be absorbed.
- It would be best if you only left when the greasy feeling has faded away.

Ingredients to look out for

There are two broad categories of sunscreens depending on the ingredients used

Physical sunscreens

- Oxybenzone
- Mineral-based: zinc oxide and titanium oxide

Chemical sunscreens

- Octinoxate
- Avobenzone

The latest combinations available are

- Tinted sunscreens (tend to be pinkish, these can also help hide spots)
- Antioxidant properties
- High SPF (suitable for sports, outdoor activities, swimming)

Treatment

Chapter 4

Chapter 4

Treatment

There's often a debate about when the right time to start treatment is. Yes, some acne clears up on its own, but it all depends on your skin type. Medication that worked for somebody else might not work for you; hence in each patient, treatment needs to be customized with a permutation and combination of topical agents, oral medication, and therapeutic modalities (physical treatment).

Treatments take time, for this same reason. As much as I tried to put 2-week deadlines on my skin clearing up for good, it never happened. In fact, it took 7 years for me to figure out the ointments, and medications that suit me.

4.1 Topical Agents

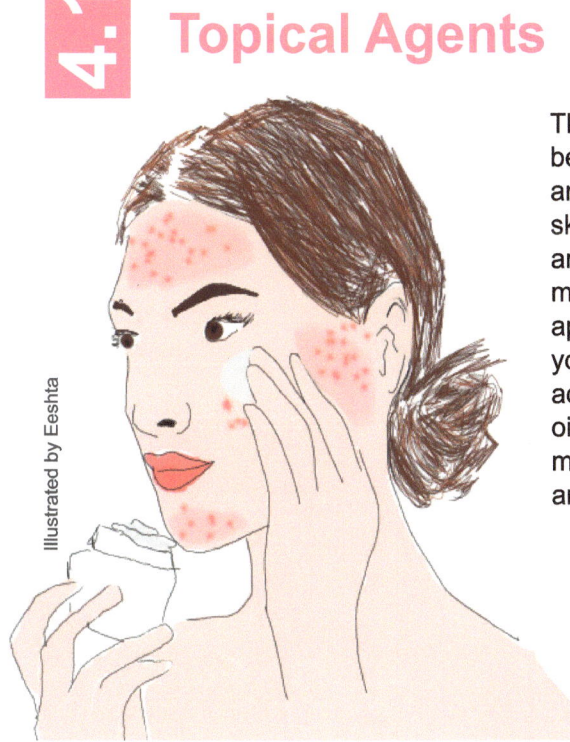

Illustrated by Eeshta

The main ingredients are benzoyl peroxide, antibiotics and retinoids. With sensitive skin types, topical agents are mixed with lotions or moisturizers, before application to avoid irritating your skin. I was often advised to combine ointments with hydrating moisturizers like Emolene, and Excela.

The main ingredients are benzoyl peroxide, antibiotics, and retinoids. With sensitive skin types, topical agents are mixed with lotions or moisturizers, before application to avoid irritating your skin. I was often advised to combine ointments with hydrating moisturizers like Emolene, and Excela.

Why I am exceedingly well acquainted with hydro nourishing moisturizer Emolene?

Emolene was the very first cream I was prescribed, which I certainly found surprising. I didn't see the point in using a moisturizer since I had extremely oily skin. I was instructed to mix benzoyl peroxide with a dollop of emolene. Later, the ointments changed from benzoyl peroxide to adapalene, retinol, clindamycin, but emolene remained constant. So, the third afternoon of every month, I'd find myself sitting in a little office, fresh out of school in my uniform, being advised on the exact volume of emolene I was supposed to combine with the acne cream. I'd then demonstrate using a bottle of standard hand lotion that I think sat at the desk for that very purpose. Suffice to say, the acne cream not having an effect always seemed to be the fault of not squeezing the right size dollop out of the emolene bottle.

Benzoyl Peroxide

Prescribed for mild to moderate acne.

How it works?
- Anti-inflammatory, comedolytic (unblocks pores), keratolytic
- Upon application, it decomposes and releases oxygen, which kills anaerobic bacteria P. acnes.
- Available in face washes, masks, lotions, ointments, creams, and gels.

Dosage: The dosage's strength varies depending on the severity of your acne and what concentration your skin can safely tolerate. Formulations are available from 2.5 to 10%.

Adverse side effects may include:
When: usually develop within the first few days of therapy, may subside with continuous use

- Shot contact therapy is advised for sensitive skin or if irritation develops.
- Cutaneous irritation
- Burning sensation
- Redness
- Bleaching of clothes, hair, and bed linen

Retinoids

- Prescribed for moderate to severe acne and mild-moderate inflammatory acne.
- Popular first-line treatment
- Family of compounds comprising vitamin A (Retinol) and its natural derivatives.

How it works?
- Regularizes abnormal keratinizations
  Unclogs blocked pores
- Work synergistically with other topical antibiotics, letting them enter pores and kill P.acnes bacteria.

Formulations available in order of decreasing potency:
- Tretinoin
- Adapalene
- Tazarotene
- Alitretinoin
- Bexarotene

These come in cream, gel, and liquid forms. Adapalene is much better tolerated than other retinoids and is the first to be prescribed. However, it depends on which compound suits you. For me, tretinoin was the best agent.

Adverse side effects may include:
- Excessive dryness of the skin
- Skin redness, scaling of the skin
- Burning

Chapter 4: Treatment

Antibiotics

Acne is not an infection, hence antibiotics will not cure it. However, they are great at quickly clearing breakouts. Clindamycin is my go-to cream when dealing with a sudden breakout of multiple tiny rash-like pimples. Popular antibiotics include clindamycin, erythromycin either used alone or together. Zinc, niacinamide are often used as co-ingredients with pure clindamycin.

How they work?
- Inhibit the growth of P.acnes bacteria on the surface of the skin and follicles.
- Reduce inflammation

Formulations:
Both available in the range of 1-4%

Adverse side effects:
Like with other agents, redness, peeling, itching, burning sensation, dryness.

Newer Topical Agents
- Salicylic Acid
- Azelaic acid (10-20% gel or cream): fruit acid, very mild, perfect for sensitive skin
- Lactic Acid
- Tea tree oil (5%): natural anti-bacterial and anti-inflammatory agent
- Picolinic acid (gel-10%)
- Dapsone Gel (5%)

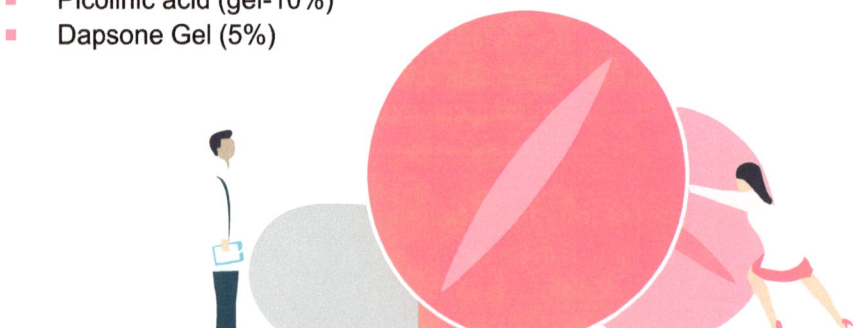

Chapter 4: Treatment

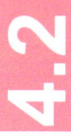

4.2 Oral Drugs

Topical treatments will almost always be supplemented with oral medications to have maximum benefit.

Antibiotics
- Most commonly prescribed since they start working instantly and effect can be seen within weeks, unlike others.
- Doxycycline, minocycline and azithromycin are the most common forms.

Others include:
- Tetracycline
- Erythromycin
- Lymecycline

My first treatment involved 2 weeks of doxycycline followed by a 2-week treatment of minocycline which greatly helped in getting rid of a particularly persistent breakout. However, these are not a permanent solution at curbing acne.

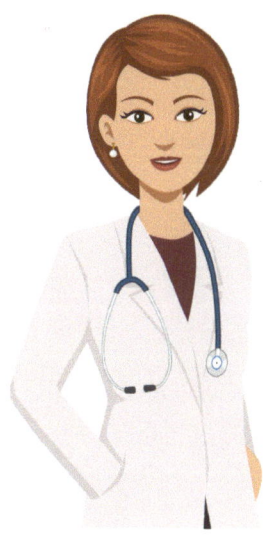

Dr. Parul Khot says:

When giving oral antibiotics, the most common issue is developing resistance.
To optimize oral therapy, only non-antibiotic topical formulations can be administered with them. The following points are adhered to:
Antibiotic monotherapy or antibiotics alone are never given alone with topical retinoids.
Benzoyl Peroxide is limited to a maximum of 3-4 months.
If retreatment is needed, as far as possible, the same antibiotic should be taken.

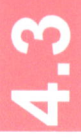 4.3 Oral Isotretinoin

When is it prescribed?
- Used for moderate to severe acne,
- Persistent acne that is not responding to conventional therapies, and oral antibiotics.
- In cases of physical scarring
- When acne has severe psychological consequences

Timing
- Unlike antibiotics, where effects are almost instantaneous, it takes at least a month to see any visible changes.
- Generally prescribed for 3-4 months.

It is commonly considered a 'Cure-all,' and is a potent drug; hence the following tests have to be conducted to ensure patients can take it:
- Baseline blood levels, a liver profile is mandatory
- Negative pregnancy test: the patient must not be pregnant at the time of taking and for six months after
- Monthly monitoring is essential to ensure the drug is not affecting body functioning.

Adverse side effects may include
(Typically start after 3-4 weeks of taking the drug and get accumulated further on)
- Headache
- Dryness of lips and eyes
- Muscle ache
- Most side effects are temporary and resolve after discontinuing the drug.

Newer formulations include micronized isotroin: improved efficacy and reduced irritancy due to microsphere technology.

4.4 Hormonal Therapy

Acne is linked to an increase in the circulation of hormones called androgens in both men and women. However, in women, hormone levels fluctuate every month with the menstrual cycle and can result in cyclical changes in acne symptoms. An increase in acne is usually observed 7-10 days before menstruation. Except for corticosteroids, hormonal therapy is reserved solely for women.

When is it necessary?
It is needed in female patients with severe oiliness, patients exhibiting androgenic hyperplasia (male pattern baldness), and SAHA syndrome (seboria, acne, alopecia).

How it works?
Prevent the effects of androgens on sebaceous glands, and follicular keratinocytes.

Types of hormonal therapy
- Oral Contraceptives
- Estrogens and progesterone decrease the level of circulating androgens.

FDA approved androgen blockers:
- Ethinylestradiol and Spironolactone are primary steroid androgen blockers. They block hormones from binding to sebaceous glands and prevent stimulation of oil production.
- CPA (strictly recommended for female patients)
- Cyproterone acetate is used in combination with ethinylestradiol as the first choice for oral hormonal therapy.

In all cases, the degree of reduction in seborrhea is drug and dose dependent.

Natural adjuvant therapies
- Kiwi extract
- Cinnamon and fenugreek extract
- Myo-inositol (vitamin B complex)

4.5 Physical Modalities in Treating Acne

Acne Removal

Comedone extraction: Mechanical removal of blackheads and whiteheads by a needle or a medical instrument.

Word of Caution: Only to be performed by a dermatologist. An incomplete extraction, refilling, tissue damage can occur if self-handled or performed at a salon.

Deep Inflammatory lesions: Pustules can be aspirated, or an intralesional steroid can be injected at the site of active skin infection.

Fruit Acid Peels

Many chemical peel options are available, derived from natural sources, including sugarcane, milk, almonds, and yeast. Popular peels are salicylic acid, glycolic acid, mandalic acid, trichloroacetic acid, and retinoic acid in various combinations and at different concentrations.

How it works?
- Peels are used as treatment options for inflamed acne.
- Reduce and subside acne
- Reduce marks, heals scars and skin
- Exfoliates skin

Fruit acid peels are by far the most popular as well as the mildest forms of treatment. However, again there is no one fit for all. I had a glycolic acid peel done, and promptly woke up the next day, with a fresh break out.

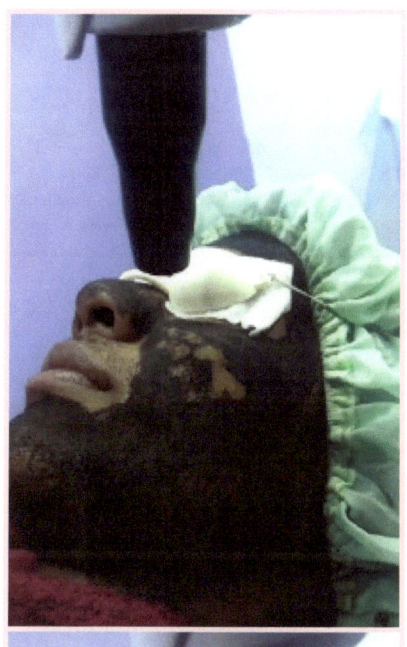

Lasers

Lasers and light treatments are the latest technology available and are extremely popular in treating inflamed acne, as well as clearing dark marks left behind by acne.

There are different laser treatments, for treating blackheads, whiteheads, acne cysts, nodules and scars. Sun protection is absolutely essential before and after treatment. More than one treatment is required for long term improvement.

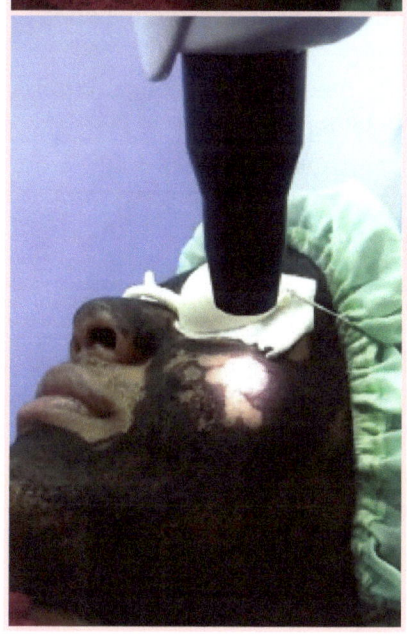

Carbon Laser Treatment

Chapter 4: Treatment

4.6 Treatment of Scars

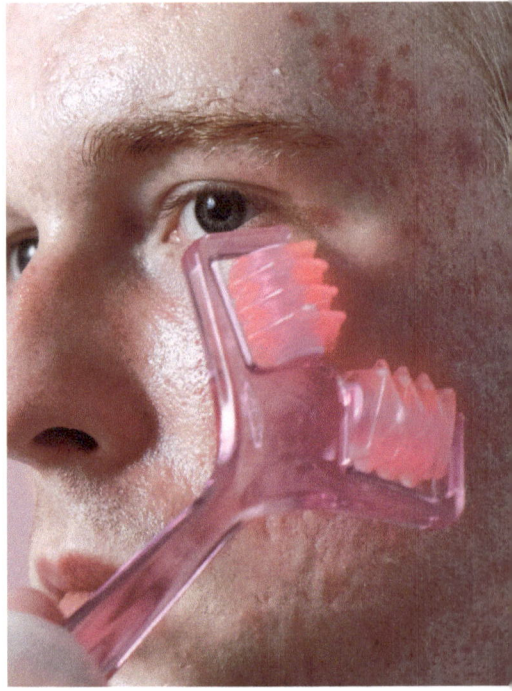

Atrophic scars (depressed)

- Punch excision and suturing
- Laser resurfacing with radiofrequency carbon dioxide lasers (ablative)
- Chemical peels
- Platelet-rich plasma
- Derma roller
- TCA cross
- Micro-needling Radiofrequency
- Fillers (Hyaluronic acid is injected under the scar to elevate it after performing subcutaneous incisional surgery).
- Subcision is a surgical procedure performed involving a hypodermic needle used to break strands that are tethering the scar to the underlying tissue.

Hypertrophic Scars (elevated)

- Intralesional steroid injection
- Surgical excision: Removal of scar tissue using a scalpel or another medical instrument.
- Cryotherapy: Localized application of freezing temperatures to destroy abnormal tissue, uses needle-like guiding device and liquid nitrogen or argon to create intense cold.

Acne and Diet

Chapter 5

Acne fighting foods

Acne causing foods

Chapter 5

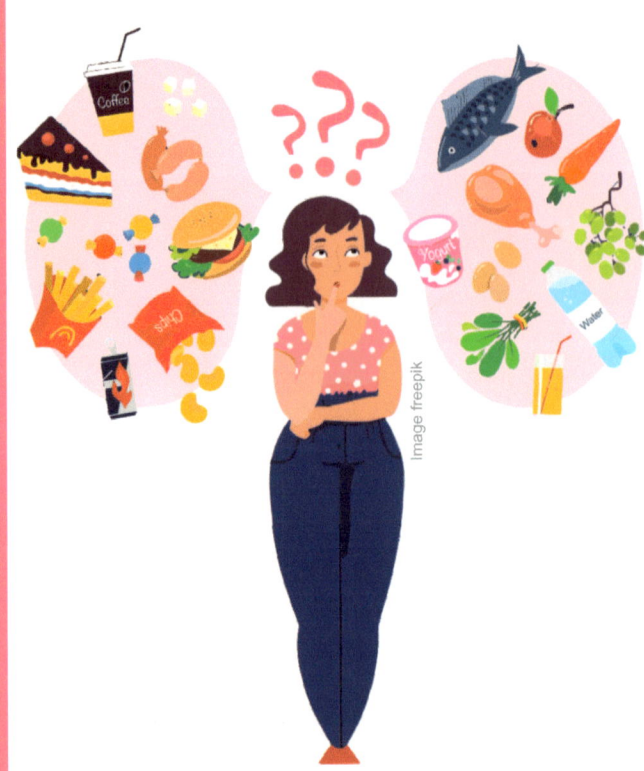

Image freepik

Acne and Diet

There's no denying that proper nutrition and a balanced diet have an extremely crucial role to play in your overall health. I'm sure we've all heard the cautionary tales of straying far away from stacks of chocolate and cheese-filled foods when first showing signs of oily acne-prone skin.

Yet, foods alone cannot cause or eliminate your acne; however, they might trigger it and exacerbate its severity. Everyone's body type and tolerances are different; hence the exact foods and ingredients that might provoke acne will differ.

The scientific community is certainly at odds with determining which food groups might be beneficial, and the mechanism behind their importance. While putting this together, I found all sorts of contradicting sources; the following groups are, however, by and large considered to be essential players in mediating acne:

Acne fighting foods

Minerals like Zinc

- A direct correlation has been seen between declining levels of zinc and increasing severity of acne.
- As a mineral, zinc regulates metabolism, supports the immune system, and controls sebum production by lowering androgens' levels.
- It also has anti-inflammatory properties and destroys acne-causing bacteria.
- Eating food sources rich in zinc helps in controlling acne. Generally, meats are rich in zinc, and supplementation can also be given as an option.

Vitamin A and E

- Fat-soluble (lipophilic)
- Low levels of these vitamins are linked to severe inflammatory acne types, pustules, cysts, and nodules.
- Failing levels of Vitamin A lead to the growth of sebaceous glands, increased sebum secretion, and P.acnes reproduction.
- Similarly, Vitamin E is anti-inflammatory, boosts your immune system, and helps with cell regeneration.
- Sunflower oil, almonds, hazelnuts
- Supplementation for both can be prescribed if they aren't part of your diet.

Antioxidants and Omega 3 Fatty Acids

Antioxidants are found in Vitamins A, C, and E.
- They are nutrients that eliminate free radicals in the body.
- Free radicals are unstable molecules that can damage healthy cells.
- Free radical skin damage is caused by pollution, UV rays, stress, and insufficient sleep.
- Both antioxidants and omega-three fatty acids neutralize damaging toxins, reduce inflammation, regulate testosterone, and androgens.

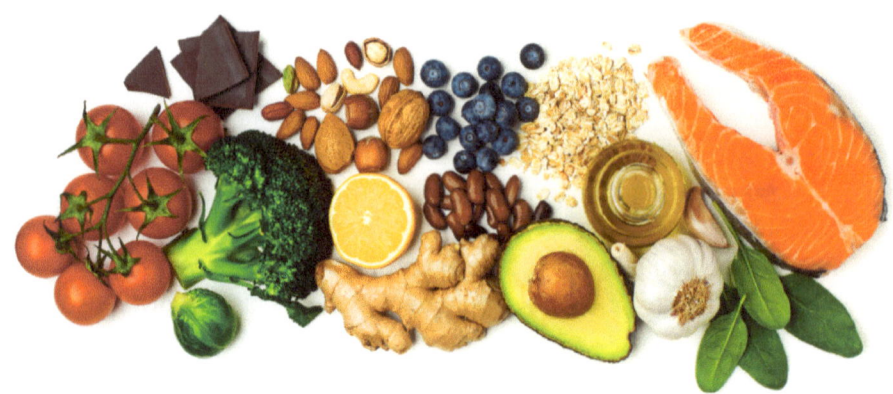

FRUITS AND VEGETABLES

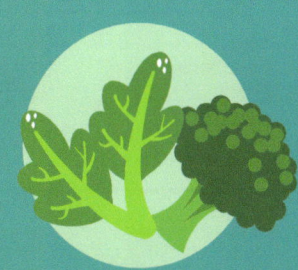

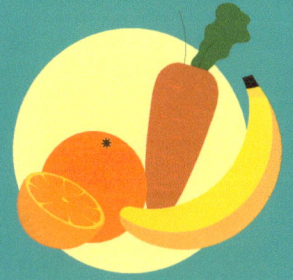

GREEN VEGETABLES

High in vitamin E, beta-carotene, fibre and a range of phytonutrients, chlorophyll Broccoli, Spinach, Kale, other dark green leafy veggies

YELLOW & ORANGE

Rich sources of Vitamin C, which protects against scarring and heals damaged irritated skin. Oranges, Bananas, Carrots, Apricot, Papaya, Sweet Potatoes

RED FRUITS

Rich in Vitamin A,C and K, acidity helps in clearing out acne and scars. Tomatoes, Strawberries, Watermelon, Apples

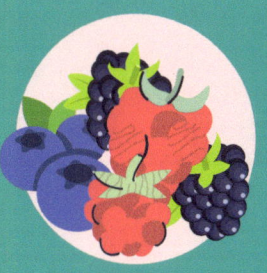

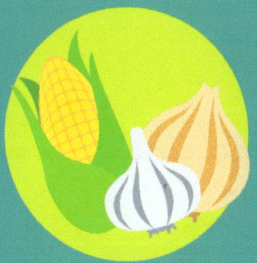

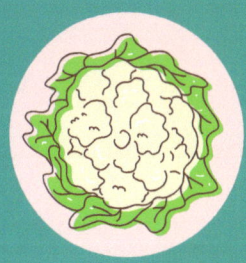

BERRIES

Rich sources of Vitamin C and antioxidants, help prevent spots and scars. Blueberries, Blackberries, Strawberries, Gooseberries, Raspberries, Cherries.

ONIONS, GARLIC AND MAIZE

Contains selenium, an antioxidant that preserves the skin's elasticity.

CAULIFLOWER

Contains amino acid 'histidine' which protects against damage from UV rays. Also a rich source of fibre, magnesium, phosphorus, Vitamin B6, C and K

OTHER FOODS

PEAS

Have a low glycemic index and are sources of Vitamin B3 (Niacinamide)

QUINOA

Contains niacinamid and compound, ecdysteroid that helps in removing scars appeared due to acne, repairs skin and minimizes irritation.

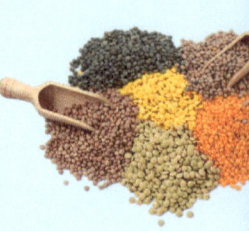

PUMPKIN SEEDS

High in Zinc and Vitamin E

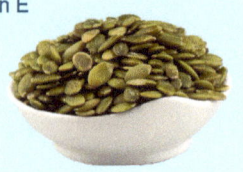

LENTILS

Contain protein and fiber, that help maintain blood sugar levels. Fluctuating levels and insulin spikes leads to acne.

WATER

Drinking at least eight glasses of water a day is the most important thing. It cleanses your skin and keeps your skin and body hydrated.

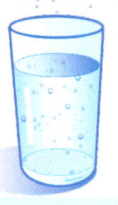

SALMON, OTHER FATTY FISH

Rich sources of Omega 3 fatty acids

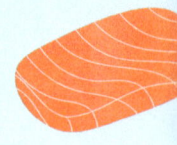

OYSTERS, CASHEWS, CHICK PEAS

Sources of zinc, fiber helps control blood sugar, which affects levels of other hormones involved in acne.

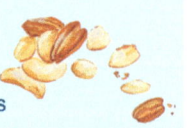

OATMEAL, CARROTS, APPLES, AND BEANS

High Fibre foods, which helps control blood sugar, which affects levels of other hormones involved in acne.

FIGS, BROWN RICE

Rich sources of magnesium that fights acne damage.

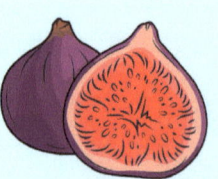

NUTS: ALMONDS, PEANUTS, CASHEWS

Rich sources of Vitamin E and selenium. Selenium increases the number of infection-fighting white blood cells in the body, while vitamin E, copper, magnesium, manganese, potassium, are all essential to skin health.

Chapter 5: Acne and Diet

Can certain foods cause acne?

During puberty, the body produces a hormone called the 'insulin-like growth factor' or IGF-1. IGF-1 increases the production of sebum and can worsen symptoms of acne.

Some foods raise IGF-1 levels; avoiding them can help in decreasing acne and preventing breakouts. Foods with high glycemic levels: these raise your blood sugar level more quickly than others. They're considered 'high-glycemic. When your blood sugar rises quickly, it causes the body to release IGF-1.

Such foods are mostly sugars and carbohydrates.

1. Breakfast foods:
    - White bread
    - Bagels
    - Sweetened breakfast cereals, cornflakes
    - Puffed rice
    - Waffles
2. Potatoes
3. Pasta and rice-based pasta
4. White rice
5. Processed and junk foods:
    - Chips, pretzels,
    - Aerated drinks and sugary sodas
    - Processed sugar cubes
    - Donuts
    - Burgers
    - French fries
    - Sweetened yogurt
6. Chocolates
    - May worsen acne symptoms because of high sugar and dairy content.
    - Dark chocolate with 100% cocoa is the best if you'd like to indulge in a chocolaty snack.

7. Greasy, fried food leads to overactive sebaceous glands.
8. Alcohol, coffee, and other food with high caffeine content can also worsen symptoms.
9. Dairy products like milk, cheese
   - Dairy is high in sugar content (lactose).
   - However, the primary issue is animal-based proteins present in dairy products and specific growth hormones added to cow and buffalo milk.
   - People with already high levels experience an over surge and are more likely to get acne.
   - Eggs are also known to contain allergens that cause acne.

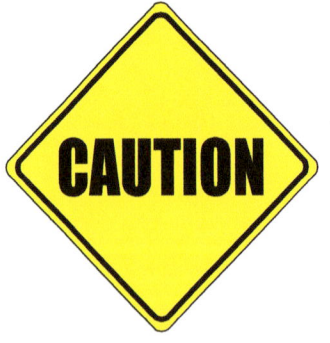

When researching different studies and articles before writing this, I was confronted with a lot of somewhat contradicting information, with various sources championing some foods. In contrast, others warned against them, and of course, I was influenced by my own experiences. The science is uncertain. There are several reasons to examine the results cautiously. Some people are wholly convinced that their diet is linked to acne breakouts and, hence, more likely to report and advise against them. Finally, there might be outliers and other factors responsible for their acne, other than nutritional sources.

ACNE CAUSING FOODS

BREAKFAST FOODS

White bread, bagels
Sweetened breakfast
cereals, cornflakes,
Puffed rice, waffles

CHOCOLATES

Dark chocolate is
rich in antioxidants
and is the best
choice when in the
mood for a
chocolate fix.

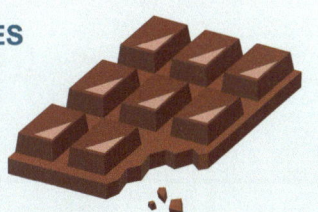

POTATOES

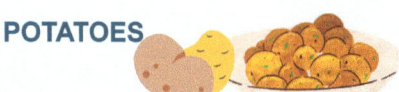

DAIRY

The primary issue is
animal-based proteins
present in dairy products
and specific growth
hormones added to cow
and buffalo milk. People
with already high levels
experience an over surge
and are more likely to get
acne. Eggs are also known to contain
allergens that cause acne.

FLOUR BASED
PASTAS

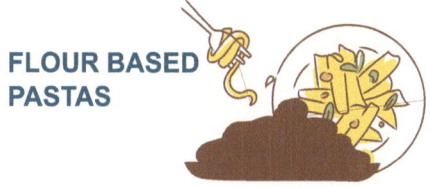

PROCESSED AND
JUNK FOODS

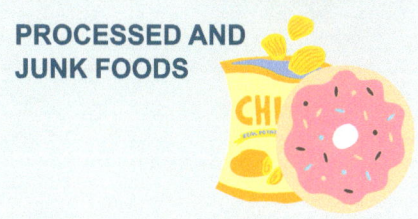

GREASY, FRIED FOOD,
CARBONATED
DRINKS

WHITE RICE

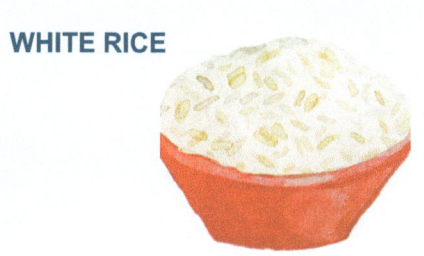

ALCOHOL, OTHER
CAFFEINATED DRINKS

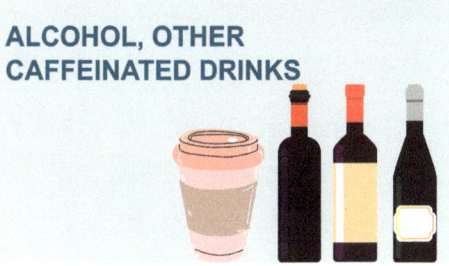

Chapter 5: Acne and Diet

Dr. Parul Khot says:

Putting together an anti-acne diet. It can be hard to know which foods to eat and which to avoid when dealing with acne but following our good food list would be a good idea.

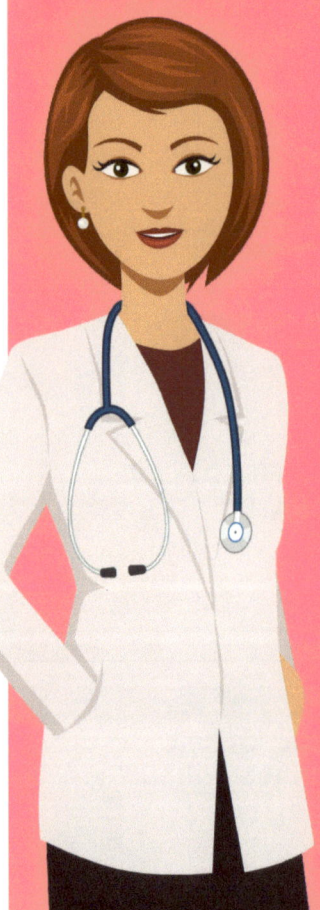

Keeping a food diary can help you identify the triggers for your acne breakouts.

Log in every meal, snack, and the severity of acne that develops each day.

- Continue this for at least a few weeks or longer.

- Have it reviewed by your dermatologist when you go for a follow-up, and then you can implement the necessary dietary changes?

- Does any food seem to worsen your breakouts? Try removing it from your diet for a week, a month? What happens then?

- Remember, be patient. After changing your diet, it can take up to 12 weeks for a dietary change to take effect.

Chapter 5: Acne and Diet

Associated Features

Chapter 6

Syndromes

Stress

Cosmetics

Chapter 6

Associated features

Sometimes, acne can be a marker or symptomatic of internal diseases and syndromes like PCOS, SAHA, and HAIR-AN. These share many similar characteristics, and symptoms including acne, increased weight gain; they are related to issues with hormonal pathways, hence seen frequently in women.

Remember that although not curable, they are treatable and can be kept under control. The reasons for their development and exact details of their pathogenesis have not yet been confirmed, but here's a quick brief:

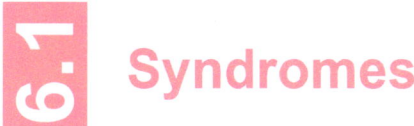 **Syndromes**

SAHA
SAHA is a medical syndrome characterized by seborrhea, acne, hirsutism, and alopecia. It is frequently associated with polycystic ovary syndrome, cystic mastitis, obesity, and infertility.

HAIR-AN
An acronym for an unusual multisystem disorder in women that consists of hyperandrogenism (HA), insulin resistance (IR), and acanthosis nigricans (AN). Acanthosis nigricans is a condition that results in the development of dark pigmented underarms, groin, side of the neck, and face.

PCOS - Polycystic ovarian syndrome
It is a hormonal disorder common among women of reproductive age of 15-40. Women's ovaries produce hormones, estrogen, and progesterone, leading to irregular and prolonged menstrual cycles.

Symptoms

- Excess levels of male hormones androgens
- Obesity, acne, oily skin, infertility
- Dark patches of skin in folds and creases
- Depression
- Loss of hair and baldness
- Excess growth of hair on face and body

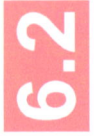 # Stress

The age-old question revolving around 'the chicken and the egg' has resulted in a great debate, still yet to be resolved. Why is this relevant? Well, because 'Acne' and 'Stress' share a similar past, a repeating cycle of cause and effect that has them closely interlinked.

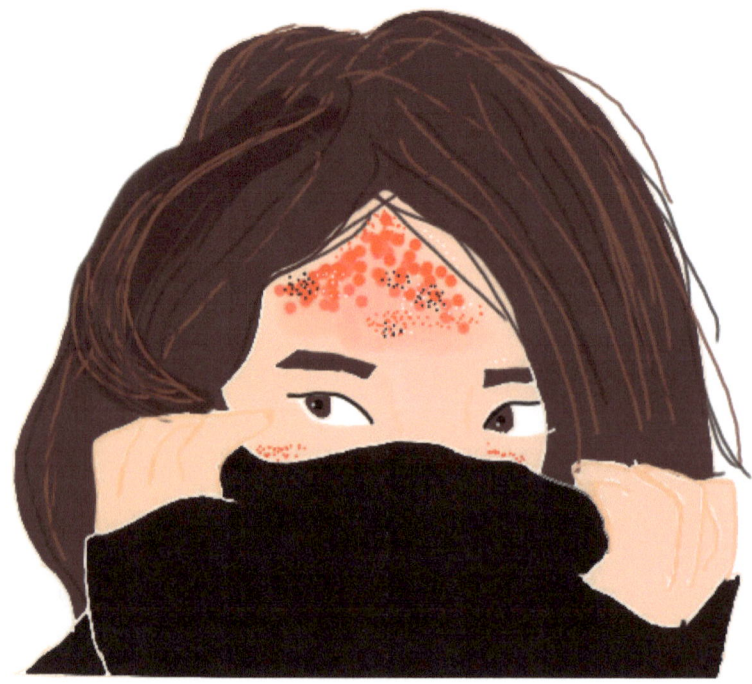

Illustrated by Eeshta

Chapter 6: Associated Features

Stress is a major trigger for acne, and acne breakouts are definitely stressors. Everyone's had the pre-'presentation, picture day, exam' pimple at least once, or if you're like me, it's just a recurring occurrence whenever stressful situations pop up. Acne might seem like a disorder confined to the surface of your skin, but its onset has a definite link to your psychological state of being.

The relationship between stress and physical appearance is affected by complex interactions in the body. There is proven research that establishes that stress triggers hormonal changes leading to acne formation in people prone to pimples.

Acute stress can lead to sudden aggravation of acne. Chronic stress drives up oil production and results in flares of resistant acne. It also interferes with the duration and resolution of breakouts.

- Healing slows down, breakouts last longer
- Increases in severity, pimples are resistant to treatment
- More likely to result in scarring

Apart from controlling biological mechanisms, stress influences our responses manifesting in behavioural signs like
- 'Stress-eating'- consuming large quantities of food, particularly chocolate, oily, greasy, processed items.
- Alternatively, forgetting to take meals regularly.
- Drinking more coffee and caffeinated drinks.
- Alcohol consumption
- Nervous habits: an increase in nerve signalling that causes you to touch your skin more frequently, aggressively pick at pimples.
- Cognitive signs: negative thoughts, worrying, anxiety, poor decision making, lack of ability to focus.

Seeing a dermatologist is the best way to determine an acne management plan and deal with your acne before a stressful situation. If you're not sure whether stress is triggering your acne breakouts, try and keep a record of stressful events and see if your acne is flaring up at the same time.

Chapter 6: Associated Features

Stress and acne interact in a harmful cycle:

The world is driven by appearances. You only see yourself in light of your flaws. Any imperfections or blemishes detract from the picture-perfect front you're required to present. Acne negatively impacts the quality of life and your emotional health, taking a toll on more than just your physical appearance; the widespread social stigma surrounding acne doesn't help.

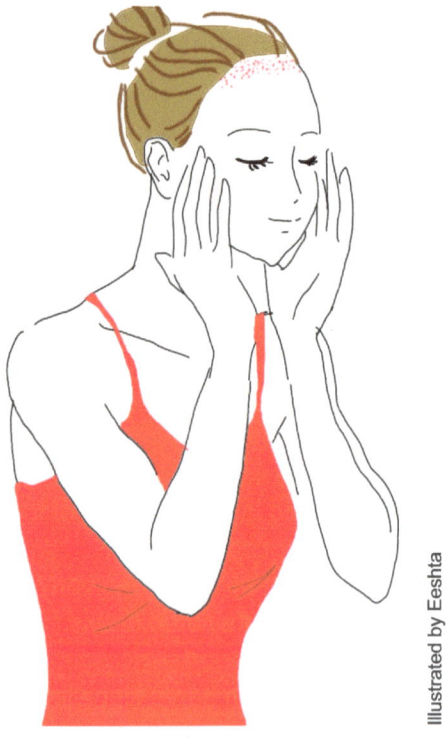

Illustrated by Eeshta

People with imperfect skin are poorly portrayed in (if they are even represented in the first place) advertising campaigns, social media, and pop culture. This often leads to alienation, the false opinion that what you're going through is something other than entirely normal, and not your fault. The most harmful are advertisements for skincare products, some of which equate with clear skin to be well behaved, responsible, and have proper hygiene habits. You do not have control over the type of skin you were born with. Some people have acne-prone skin; others do not.

Chapter 6: Associated Features

There are pernicious psychological consequences that stem from this societal stigma, including:

- General insecurity
- Low self-esteem
- Inferiority complex
- Anxiety
- Depression
- Maladjustments

Presenting itself in the already tumultuous teenage years can be one of the most significant impediments to relationship building and self-esteem. Loss of self-confidence, especially if it provokes taunts, comments from peers.

The main fear is one of negative appraisal, perceptions by others, leading to a tendency to avoid making eye contact, covering the face with hair, and truncal acne even influences clothing choices and avoidance of certain activities like swimming for fear of exposing blemished skin.

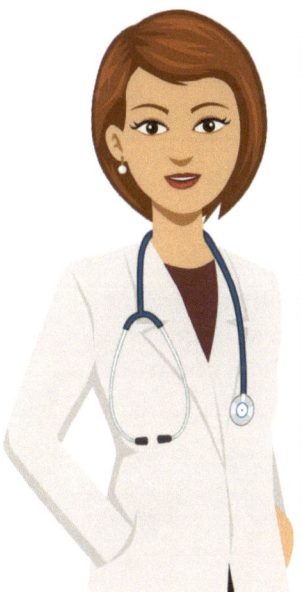

Dr. Parul Khot says:

What makes matters worse is that acne is rarely ever resolved instantaneously; it's a long term disorder, with recurrences, relapses, resistance. Patients usually lose patience, leading to many emotional complications ranging from as low as insecurity to complete social withdrawal. It's desperately important to see a dermatologist so you can get professional holistic care and manage your acne before it has long-lasting effects on your mental health.

Chapter 6: Associated Features

Help comes in many forms.
Ways to combat stress:

Acne Excoriee

Sometimes, when you're worried and embarrassed about your skin, every little blemish is amplified, and there's an extreme urge to pick at it compulsively; it's often impossible to stop. And eventually, it becomes an ingrained habit, a reflex action when you're worried, tense, or have nothing else to do with your hands.
Stress acne cannot be eliminated until you manage your stress levels.

Yoga

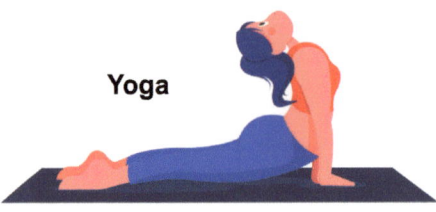

Meditation

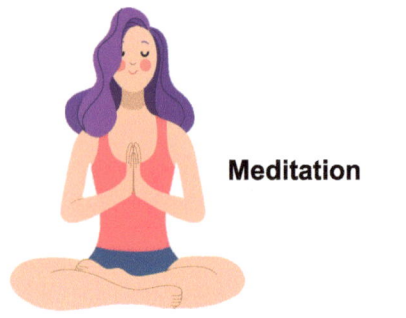

A walk

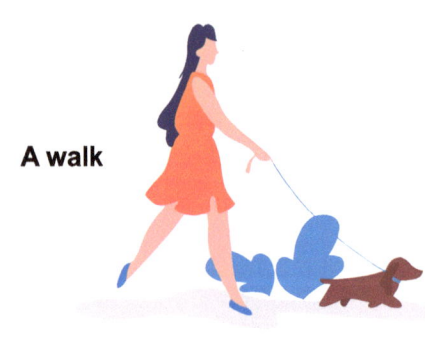

Me-time

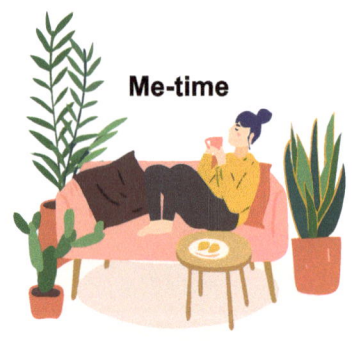

Image freepik

Spa day

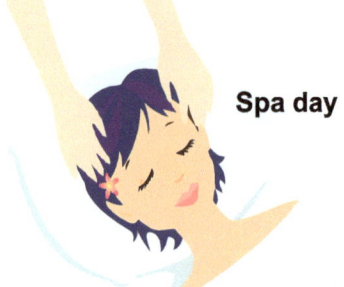

Talk with a friend or therapist, someone you trust

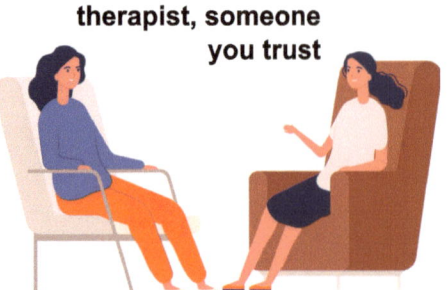

Chapter 6: Associated Features

6.3 Cosmetics

When I was going through a particularly rough flare up at 13, I carefully sneaked out some foundation from my mother's cabinet. I padded it gently onto my face before heading out. Once or twice, even to school.

When she found out, my mother was naturally livid, and we had a whole spat about it. I understand the impulse now, but it was entirely the wrong way to go about it.

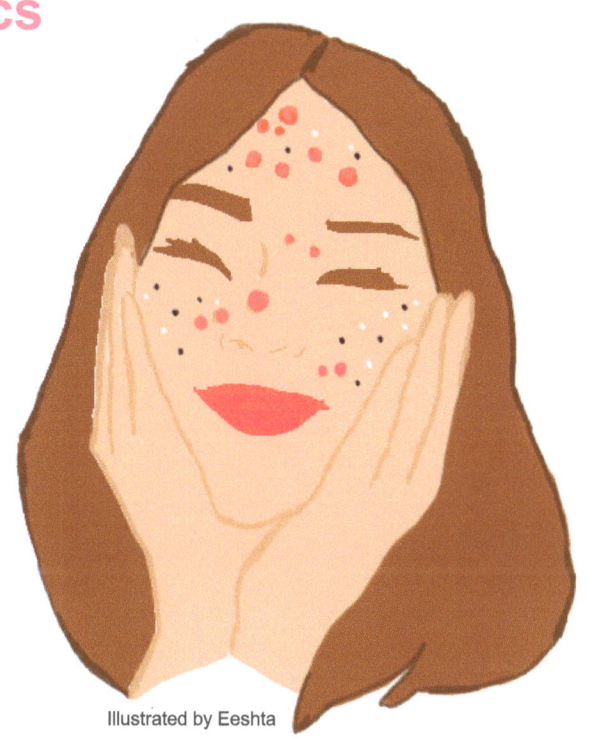

Illustrated by Eeshta

Most makeup does not cause acne, but certain ingredients can clog pores, helping P.acnes grow and trigger flare-ups in acne-prone skin.

There's no denying that covering acne lesions, marks, and scars goes a long way in helping you feel more comfortable in your skin, reignite confidence levels and boost self-esteem. I always felt way surer of myself with my skin feeling unblemished and clear, protected by a trusty concealer.

However, using the wrong products, or not going about in the right way, can lead to a never-ending cycle of breakouts and leave you feeling much worse.

COSMETICS

SAFEST BRANDS TO USE

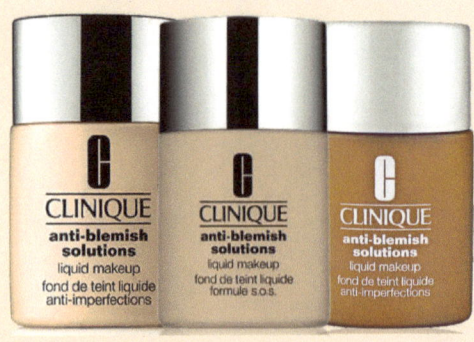

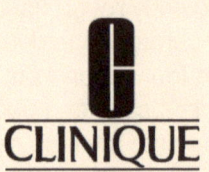

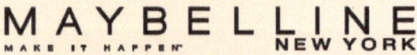

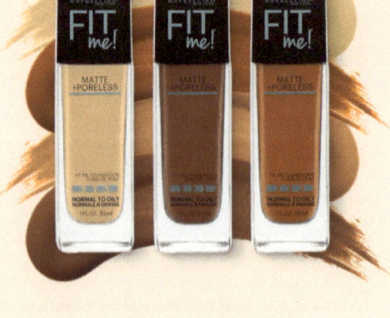

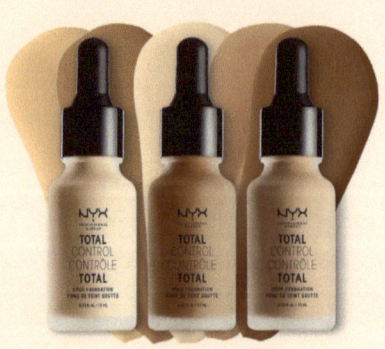

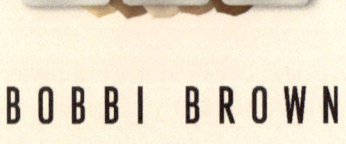

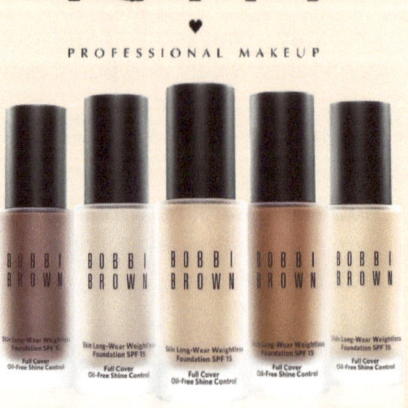

Chapter 6: Associated Features

How do you find the right formulation for your skin?

There are a LOT of products out there, claiming to cover even the most resistant acne, yet most appear dry, caky, accentuating pimples and scars rather than concealing them.

Make sure you're using a moisturizer before applying primer, foundation, and concealer. For heavy makeup, a toner is also a must.

Look for the following when purchasing foundations and concealers:
- Noncomedogenic
- Shine-free
- Matte
- Liquid
- Lightweight
- Oil-free
- Hydrating foundation

If you can, try products that use micro-clear technology. They contain a unique blend of salicylic acid that unclogs pores and dissolves them while concealing existing lesions and scars.

MINERAL MAKEUP is the latest trend that is making the rounds. It is free of:
- Parabens
- Fillers
- Binders
- Synthetic chemicals

Primary Ingredients:
Zinc oxide, iron oxides, titanium dioxide, organic oils

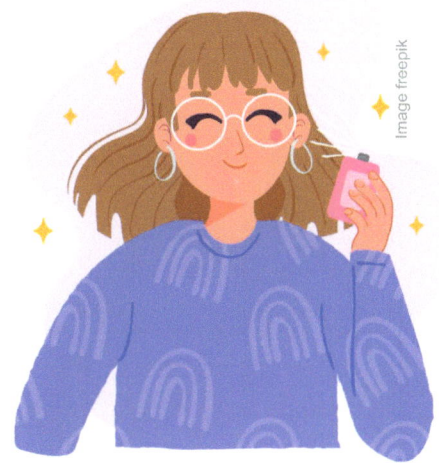

Image freepik

Chapter 6: Associated Features

Whichever products you choose, the most important thing to do is to remove them from your skin at the end of the day. Do not keep cosmetics on while sleeping. This will irritate your skin, and allow the makeup to sink deep into your pores, blocking them and causing breakouts.

Cleansers or removers ensure that your pores do not get clogged.

Illustrated by Eeshta

Chapter 6: Associated Features

REMOVERS
SAFEST BRANDS TO USE

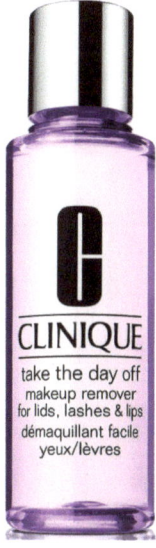 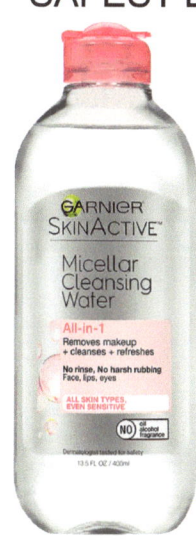 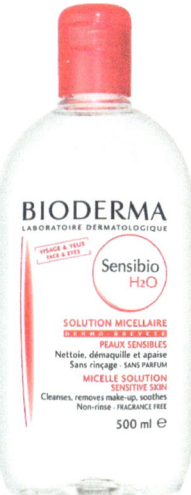 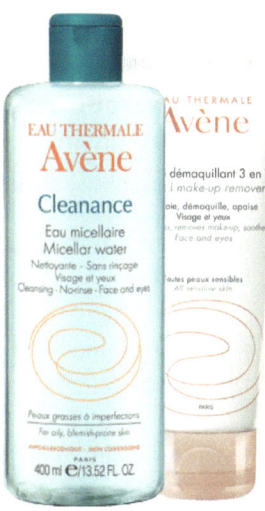

INGREDIENTS TO LOOK OUT FOR

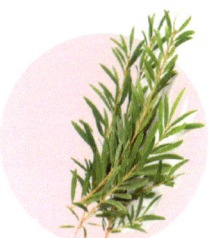

Tea tree extract

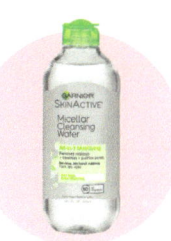

Micellar Water

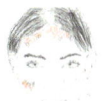

Tip: After cleansing my face of make-up, I always splash my face with ice cold water, to reduce redness, itchiness, and help cool the surface of the skin.

Micellar Water is made using purified water, moisturizers like glycerine, and mild surfactants, which are compounds used for cleansing. Removes, dirt, makeup, oil, enables cleansers to penetrate to deeper layers, extremely gentle, and promotes skin hydration.

Chapter 6: Associated Features

On the go acne care

Face Wipes and Pads are excellent alternatives to washing when on the move. They remove oil and help prevent over washing. **Fresh makeup brushes** must be used at all times.

It is a good idea to replace them every six months or so since they represent a potential nidus for infection.

PRO-TIP: Cleaning your make-up brushes

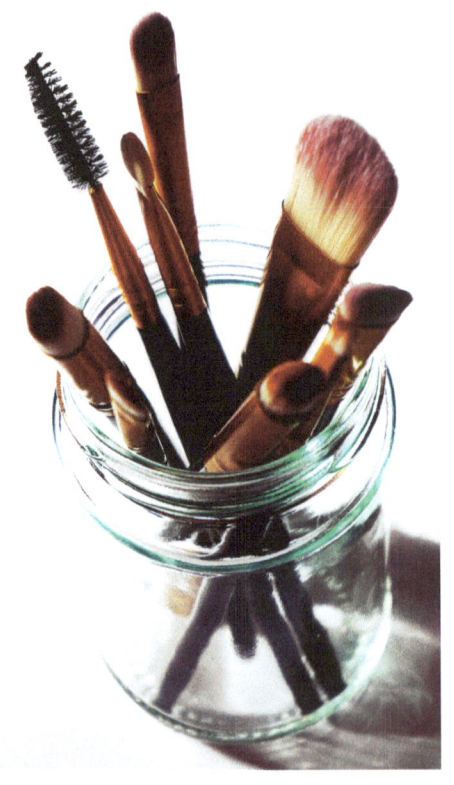

Even new, unused brushes can cause breakouts. To help reduce breakouts, it is important to remove all traces of product and dust, dirt build-up from the brush hairs. Here's a quick and easy way to thoroughly cleanse your brush.

1. Run your brushes in lukewarm water upside-down. So metal handles don't get wet.

2. Then in a bowl or glasses, prepare a solution of lukewarm water and Dettol.

3. Soak your brushes upside-down for at least an hour.

4. Gently pat dry.

5. Let the brushes dry, on tissue paper, letting the bristles hang out.

You must do this after every application, especially brushes you use for applying foundation and concealers. This ensures there is no product build-up, in the bristles.

My Guide To Clear Skin

Chapter 7

Cleansers

Treatment

Diet and Recipes

Chapter 7

My Guide to Clear Skin

When I first visited a dermatologist starting at age 11, I was given a list of instructions that felt like it was infringing on every aspect of my life. Taking facewashes to school, three different face towels for each time I washed my face, being told I had a hypersensitivity to the sun, limiting my physical activities.

And of course, the dietary restrictions: cut down on cheese, cut down on sweet pastries, chocolate. But even with the following most of the recommendations, very few of them yielded any positive results. I have used almost all ointments, gels, and quite a few oral drugs, including two isotretinoin courses. So, after seven years and a lot of ups and downs, with impromptu breakouts, I have a guide on what works for me, and I hope it helps you narrow down what works for you as well.

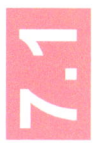 ## Cleansers and Face Washes

One of the easiest things to do when dealing with acne-prone oily skin is making sure you wash your face at least twice a day, in the morning and night. However, this is only a reference, I took this metric literally, to avoid washing my face in school and when I was out. It depends on your skin type. If you have an extremely oily skin type like me, it's important you wash your face as soon as you can feel the greasiness and oil set in. I remember trying really hard to resist from picking and scratching at my face, due to oily film attracting dust and other particles.

MY PICKS: CLEANSERS, FACE WASHES AND SCRUBS

Gently massage the face while cleansing to ensure products can unclog pores and remove impurities. Do not scrub, this will only irritate your skin.

Cleansing 101

01

The very first face wash I picked up. Gentle, water based and cheap, this face wash ensure a clean feel without drying your skin.

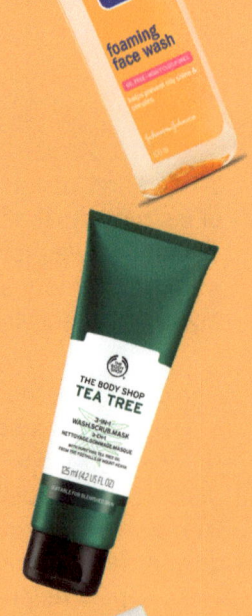

02

This scrub is absolutely perfect for oily blemished skin. It leaves you with a fresh cool feeling even after washing, without irritating your skin. After long sweaty runs, and dance routines, this scrub is the perfect addition to your end of the day cleanse.

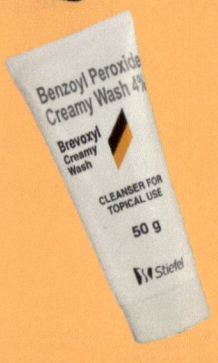

03

For very oily skin, this benzoyl peroxide creamy wash is ideal at removing oil, and grease without causing redness and inflammation.

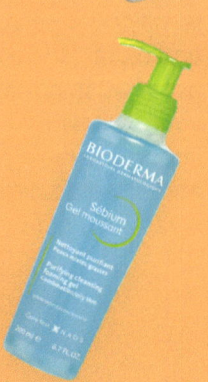

04

To avoid over cleansing my skin, I love using this face wash which is gentle and calming and helps balance harsher cleansers.

Finding a proper cleanser is the next step. I earlier mistakenly believed two things at various points: Firstly, I opted for products that were extremely gentle and calming, afraid that even the were the only ones which wouldn't irritate my sensitive skin. But these were best suited for dry skin and did little to remove oil from my face. So naturally, these really didn't help my skin.

Chastised, I went for harsher products that left my skin stinging. I mistakenly believed this was great, burning meant it was working right? The only thing it led to was excessive drying.

You have to choose a cleanser that leaving your skin feeling cleansed, but at the same time doesn't strip it of its natural moisture. These are my top picks:

Skin Stories

When I was thirteen, I visited a second dermatologist. Acne had now spread from my forehead onto my once pristine cheeks, resulting in angry red splotches that stood out glaringly against my skin, made even more prominent, since my skin reddens at the slightest exertion be it laughing, walking, or exercising.

Anyway, I was told that it was simply a question of genetics. Thick curly frizzy hair, fair sensitive skin, and having parents that had had both experienced acne, was just the holy trinity, I was doomed to have acne no matter what. This didn't go very well, understandably. But later on, I did realise that your hair can actually be a huge trigger for acne. Products including shampoos, conditioners, serums, can drip down while you're washing your hair or after, and irritate your skin.

Dandruff can also lead to acne since both are a product of excess sebum production.

Oily scalp- dandruff- grease spreads to forehead- acne breakouts

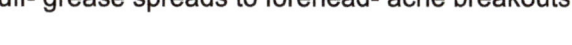

Chapter 7: My Guide To Clear Skin

Treatment

MY PICKS: TOPICAL AGENTS THAT DON'T IRRITATE SENSITIVE SKIN

01

Clindamycin is perfect for dealing with rashes, sudden breakouts.

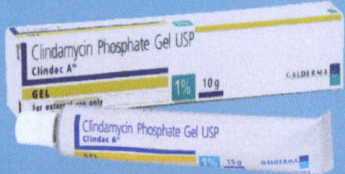

02

Atorrege AD+ Acne Spots is a product formulated by Japanese skin care company that offers a range of acne care products curated for any number of sensitive skin types, oily, acne prone, normal, combination.

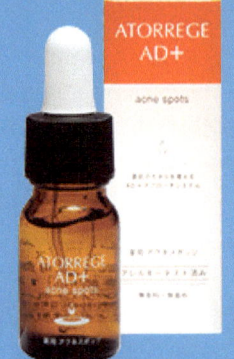

03

Formulations containing retinoid acid. However it can take some time to figure out which one works for you. I generally used a gel combining adapalene and benzoyl peroxide.

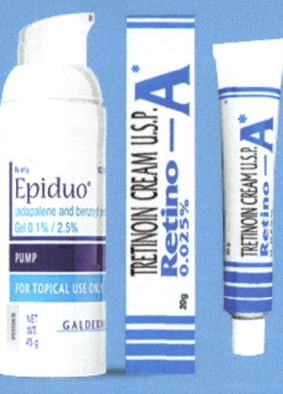

04

Fruit acid based products can work wonders. For my skin type, Salicyclic acid and Azaleic acid work the best.

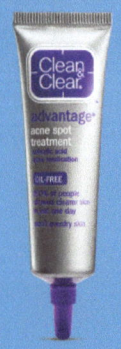
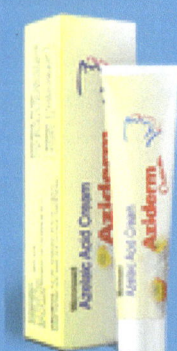

Chapter 7: My Guide To Clear Skin

7.2 Treatment

I've always been super wary of trying out just any new product, due to the violent acne flare-ups I've had over the years. It's frustrating, and well I reached a point where I would rather put nothing than deal with the consequences of trying something new. Unfortunately, the only way forward is to trial test with different treatments. Here's some that have worked for me over the years. It's always best to mix acne gels and creams with a trusted moisturizer and then slowly wean it off, if required, so that it does not irritate your skin.

Further sometimes certain commercially sold creams and ointments will have multiple active compounds working together. You might have to experiment with these individually as well to see which works for you.

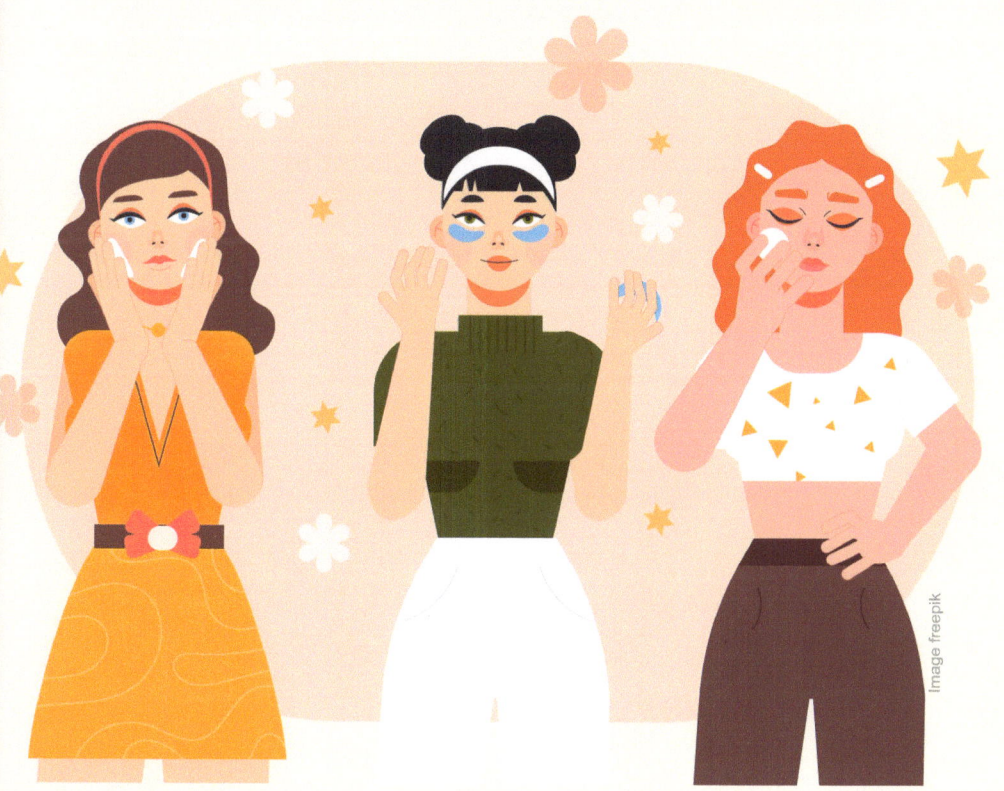

Image freepik

Chapter 7: My Guide To Clear Skin

MY PICKS: ACNE PATCHES, DANDRUFF CARE AND ALOEVERA

Other products

01

Dandruff and acne often appear together. This cooling foam cleared my forehead acne in days. Simply apply, keep it overnight, and wash in the morning if you notice pimples breakout out along your hairline, forehead and temples.

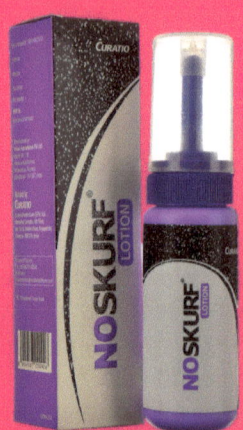

02

Acne patches were a part of my daily routine.I would wake up every morning and promptly plaster one over a troublesome whitehead. Helps clear infection, prevents you from picking at it, and even effectively hides the spot from view. It's perfect for pimples that pop up last minute, and just won't clear. I use the ones from Nexcare, but there are now a host of options available in slew of different shapes, colours and sizes.

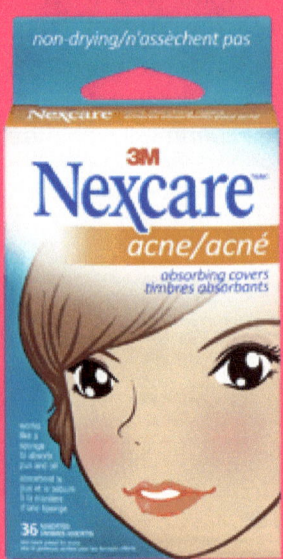

03

Aloe Vera is perfect when dealing with inflamed skin, redness and bad reactions to certain products. It has antibacterial, antioxidant and anti-inflammator properties, hence is also effective in treating acne, and reducing marks.

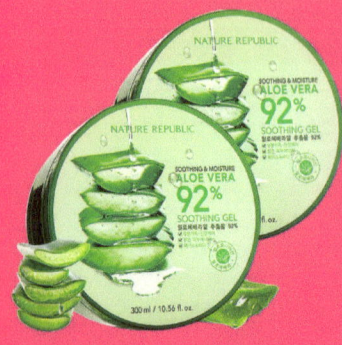

7.3 Diet

I've always been a very reluctant cook; whipping up meals in the kitchen was never really my cup of tea. But, I positively hated the meals that I had to eat instead: blanched spinach soup, papaya, and watermelon. Next came the stomach cleansers, wheat husk, strained neem juice, bitter gourd, and blood purifiers. Naturally, this just made me even more determined to sneak in packets of crisps, donuts, and, well, whatever I could manage.

Dietary correlations exist between acne and diet; high-fat, high-sugar foods promote inflammation throughout the body. Certain foods contain hormones that further contribute to the hormonal imbalance in your body. This does not mean eating a meal should have to become a dreaded activity.

Changing your dietary habits is impossible if you're not in full control of your making changes. Remember, science isn't exact; there's no way to definitely prove that diet causes acne. One of the primary reasons I grew quickly tired of following meal plans was that I couldn't really see any significant difference in my skin. Of course, I never committed to it for longer than a week without slipping up along the way, but I didn't see the point in enduring meals that I hated and still not having clear skin. I'd instead at least enjoy food and then deal with the consequences. I was mistaken. It's essential to eat a balanced antioxidant-rich diet with all food groups (lots of fruits and vegetables), but there are different forms and combinations that these can be eaten in.

If you do plan to change your diet, it has to be your decision, and with foods and recipes you like. Otherwise, it will be simply impossible to sustain in the long run. This year, I finally crossed the sacred threshold and stepped into the kitchen. I have included some quick, healthy snacks that I started making to make the transition a little easier. So the next time you feel like munching, you can do so guilt-free.

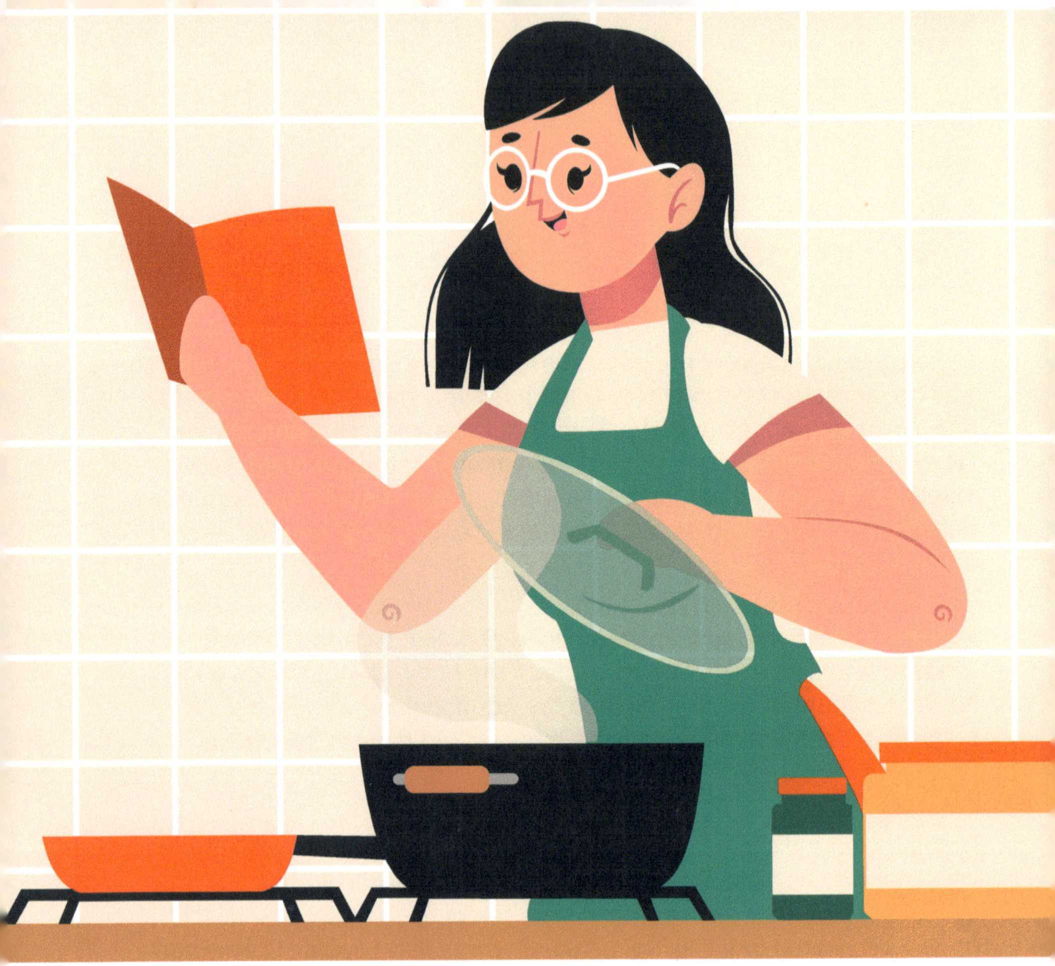

Recipe

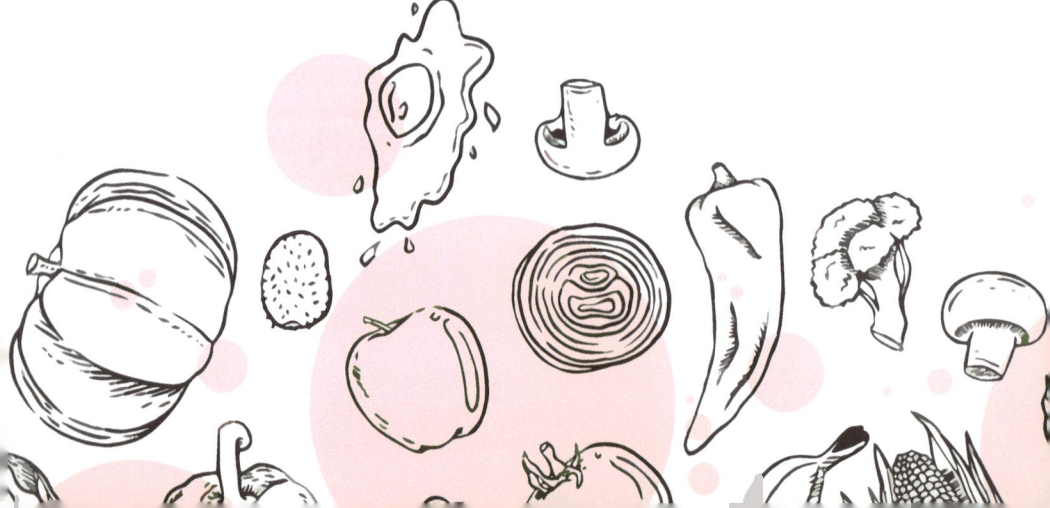

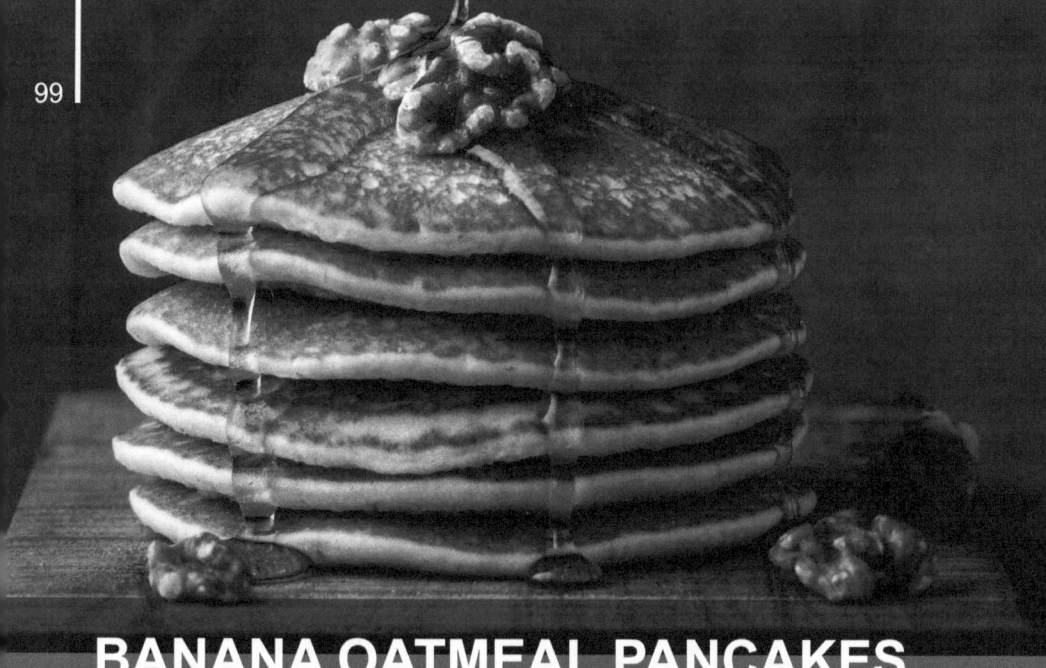

BANANA OATMEAL PANCAKES

Oats contain zinc, which has anti inflammatory
properties and helps inhibit the growth of acne
causing bacteria. They also help reduce oil production.
They're also low on the glycemic index.

Ingredients

- 2 medium ripe bananas

- 2 1/2 tablespoons white sugar
  1/2 teaspoon salt

- 2 cups oat flour

- 1 cup all-purpose flour

- 1 tablespoon baking powder

- 1 cup milk

- 1 teaspoon ground cinnamon

**PREPARATION: 10MIN
COOKING: 10 MIN
READY IN: 20 MIN**

Directions

1. Place oats in food processor,
ground until semi fine. If they form too
fine a powder, the pancakes will not
be fluffy and light. Mash bananas.
Combine ground oats, bananas and
milk, let them sit for around 10
minutes.

2. After, stir in rest of ingredients.
Brush oil in a large non-stick pan over
medium heat. Pour batter and cook
until edges are golden brown, about
2-3 minutes, flip the pancake and
cook for another 2-3 minutes. Repeat
until batter is all gone.

3. Serve with your choice of toppings.
I love maple syrup, walnuts, and
some cinnamon.

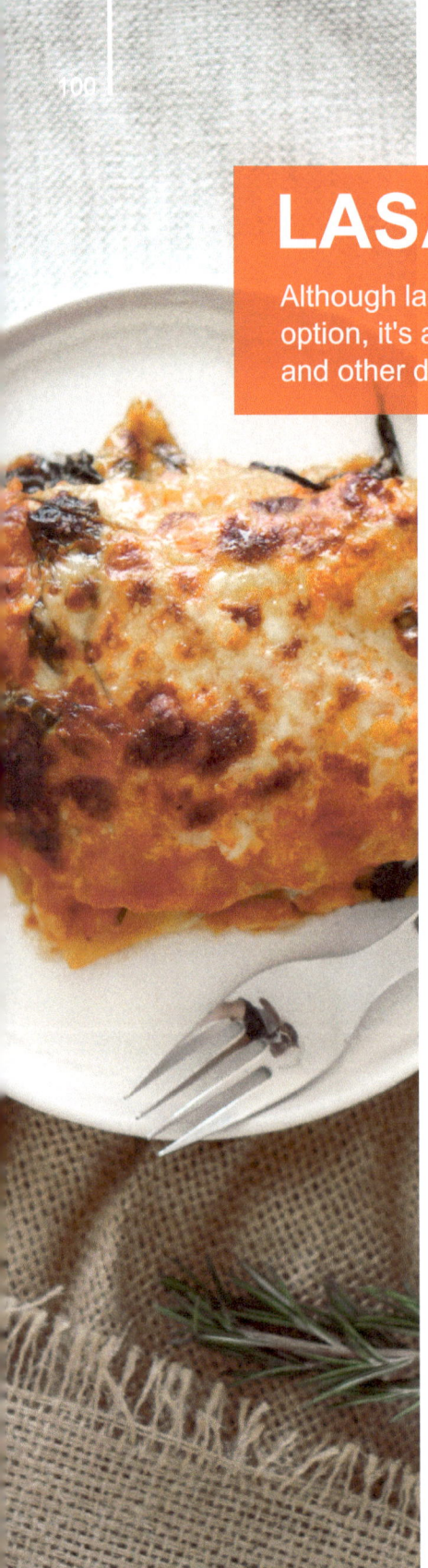

LASAGNA

Although lasagna might seem like an unhealthy option, it's a great way to eat lots of spinach, and other dark green vegetables.

The Ingredients

- 2 tablespoons butter

- 2 tablespoons extra-virgin olive oil

- 1/2 cup chopped onions

- 3 medium cloves garlic, minced (about 2 tablespoons)

- Salt and freshly ground black pepper

- Spinach chopped

- 4 tablespoons butter

- 21/2 tablespoons flour

- 3 cups whole milk

- Mozzarella cheese

- Cheddar cheese

- 5 tomatoes

- Choice of vegetables, one cup each: broccoli, bell peppers, carrots

- Whole wheat lasagna noodles

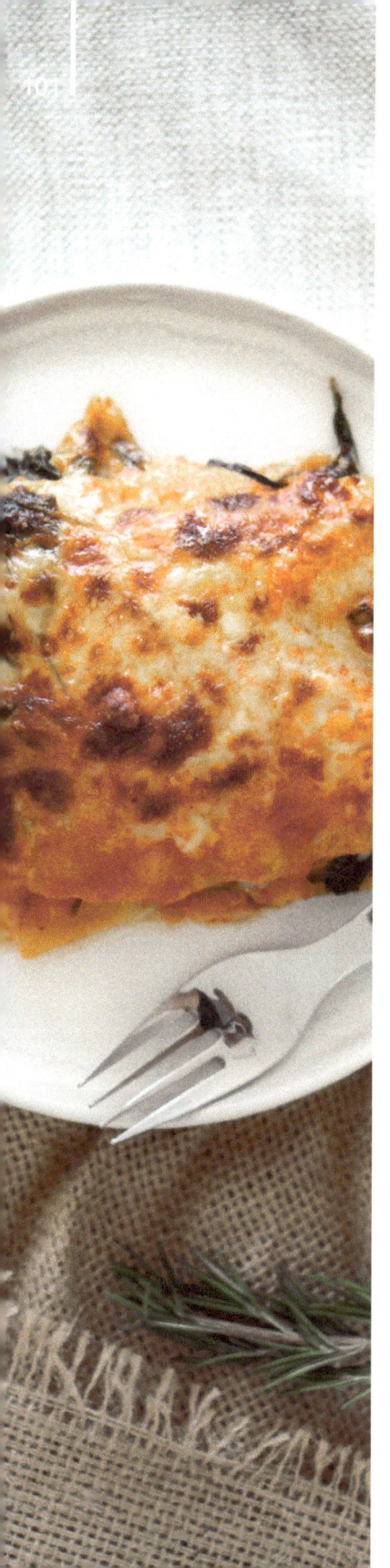

Directions

- Preheat oven to 350°F. Bring a large pot of salted boiling water to a boil and cook lasagna noodles until al dente. Carefully remove and drain.

- Red Sauce: In a pan, over medium heat, heat olive oil. Add onion and garlic and season with salt, pepper, and oregano. Add tomato paste, and a cup of water. Let the mixture cook for around 7 minutes. Add cut vegetables of your choice. I like bell peppers, broccoli, and carrots.

- When finished, stir in the cut spinach, and keep over heat for 1-2 minutes. Take off. Béchamel (White sauce): Heat butter in a over medium heat until melted. Add flour and increase heat. Cook, stirring butter and flour with a whisk until paled golden blond, about 1 minute. Whisking constantly, slowly add milk. Continue to cook, whisking frequently, until mixture comes to a boil and thickens. Remove from heat and add cheese. Whisk until smooth. Season with salt, pepper, and oregano.

- In a large baking dish, layer lasagna noodles so they overlap slightly. Spoon over a thin layer of red sauce and top with a layer of white. Sprinkle with a layer of mozzarella. Repeat, ending with mozzarella.

- Bake for around 15-20 minutes, until the layer of mozzarella starts to brown.

CREAMY FENUGREEK, GREEN PEAS CURRY

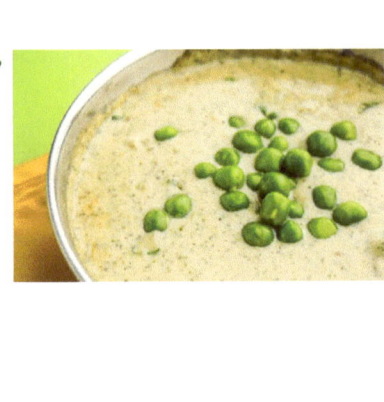

The Ingredients

- 1 big bunch of methi leaves or fenugreek, tough stems removed, washed, then finely chopped.
- 2 cups green peas
- ⅓ cup chopped onions
- ¼ cup cashews
- 1 teaspoon chopped garlic cloves
- 1 teaspoon ginger
- 1 teaspoon green chilies
- 2 green chillies, chopped
- 1 tsp cumin seeds
- 1 tbsp vegetable oil
- 1 1/4 cup milk
- 2 tbsp fresh cream

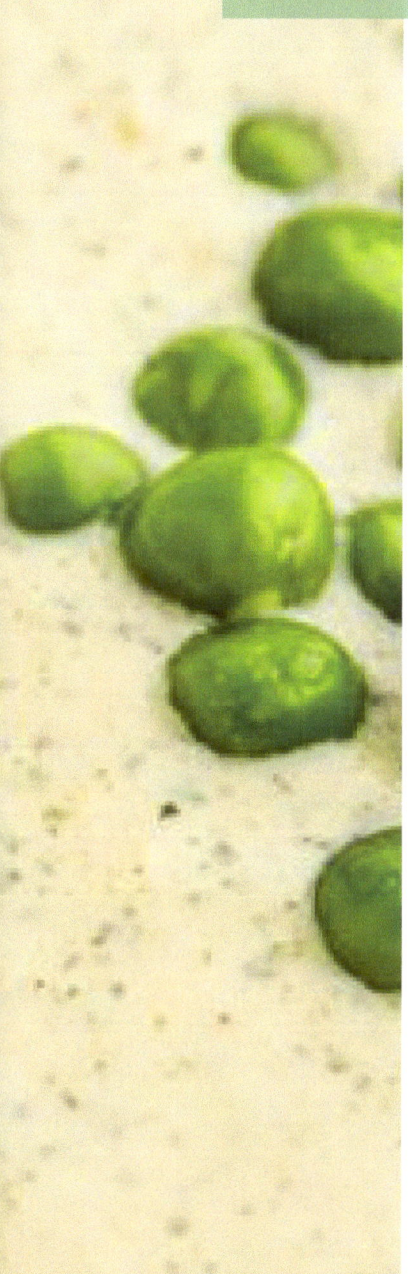

CREAMY FENUGREEK, GREEN PEAS CURRY

Directions

- In a grinder jar, add 1 teaspoon cumin seeds, ⅓ cup chopped onions, ¼ cup cashews, 1 teaspoon chopped garlic cloves, 1 teaspoon ginger and 1 teaspoon green chilies.

- Grind to a smooth paste.

- Heat some oil in a pan.

- Add the ground paste and fry the paste 6 to 7 minutes on low flame till it starts giving a fragrant aroma.

- Keep on stirring in between to avoid the paste from sticking to the pan.

- You should see oil releasing from the sides. Do not brown the paste. Add the milk and cream.

- Add a little water if it sticks to the pan. Add chopped fenugreek leaves and saute for 2 minutes.

- Then add ½ cup water in parts. Mix well and simmer for 3 to 4 minutes. Stir at intervals.

- Then add the boiled peas and cream.

- Simmer gravy for 5 to 6 minutes on a low flame. Add salt to taste. Serve hot.

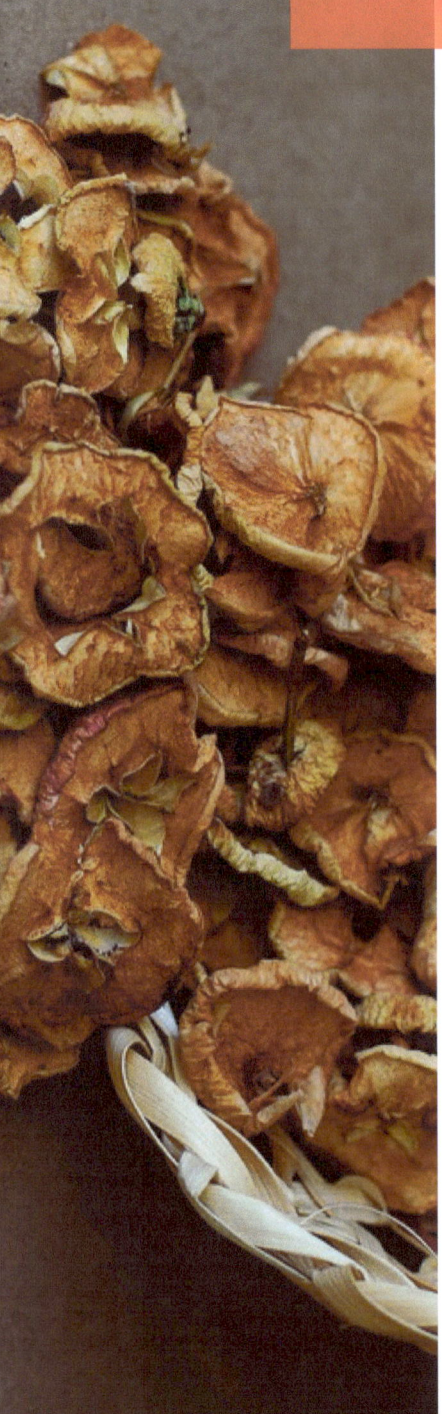

BAKED APPLE CHIPS

Prep Time: 5 minutes
Cooking time: 2 - 4 hours
Total: 4 hours 5 minutes

Directions

- Preheat oven to 200°F.

- Wash and thinly slice the apples as shown in the photos above. Spread the apple slices onto the baking pans making 1 single layer.

- Sprinkle with cinnamon and nutmeg.

- Bake for 1 hour, flip the apples over, and bake for another 1-1.5 hours.

- Turn the oven off and keep the apples inside as the oven cools down for 1 hour. This will help them get crunchy. Alternatively if you'd like them chewy, you could flip them after half an hour.

- Some apples may just be chewy and only slightly crunchy after 3 hours in the oven.

- Store them in a box for munching. They should stay for up to one week.

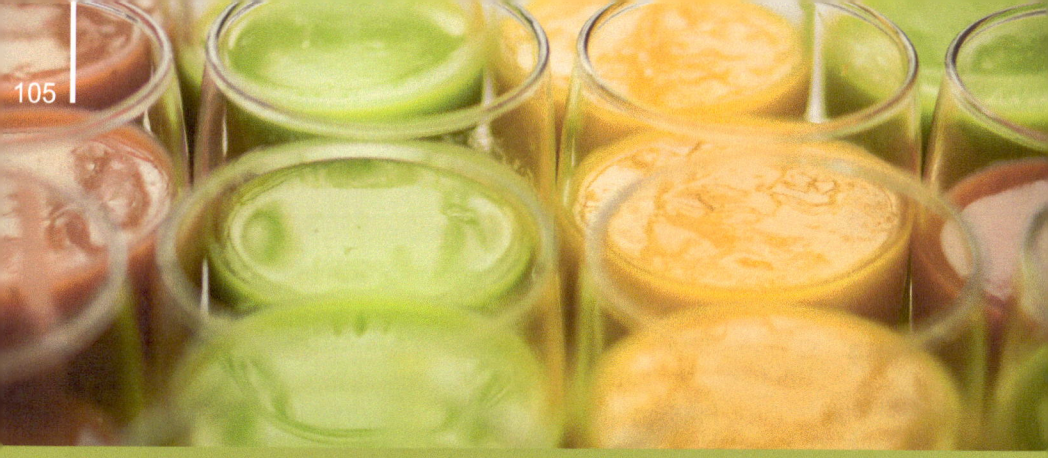

SMOOTHIES

Healthy Options

- Berry Blast: Strawberries, blueberries, raspberries
- Strawberries and Banana
- Banana and Peanut Butter
- Orange, Lemon, Spinach and Mint
- Mango, Oats, Milk, Honey
- Apple, Lemon, Ginger, Spinach
- Carrot, Orange, Apple
- Strawberries, Mint, Yoghurt
- Mango, Pineapple, Oats
- Watermelon, Mint, Lemon
- Grapes, Kale, Lemon

Directions

- 2 Cups fruits or any mix of fruits and veggies
- 1 cup liquid, milk, water, juice
- Optional: 1/2 cup yoghurt
- Place frozen fruit, liquid, and any optional add-ins into a blender.
- Blend on high until smooth. You can add more liquid depending on how thick you like your smoothie.

JUICES

Vegetables and fruits contain essential fibres and nutrients that help flush out toxins. Further, they contain antioxidants that inhibit the growth of free radicals which damage body cells. Some essential juices to incorporate in your diet are: watermelon, apple, ginger lemon, papaya, orange, tomato and pomegranate.

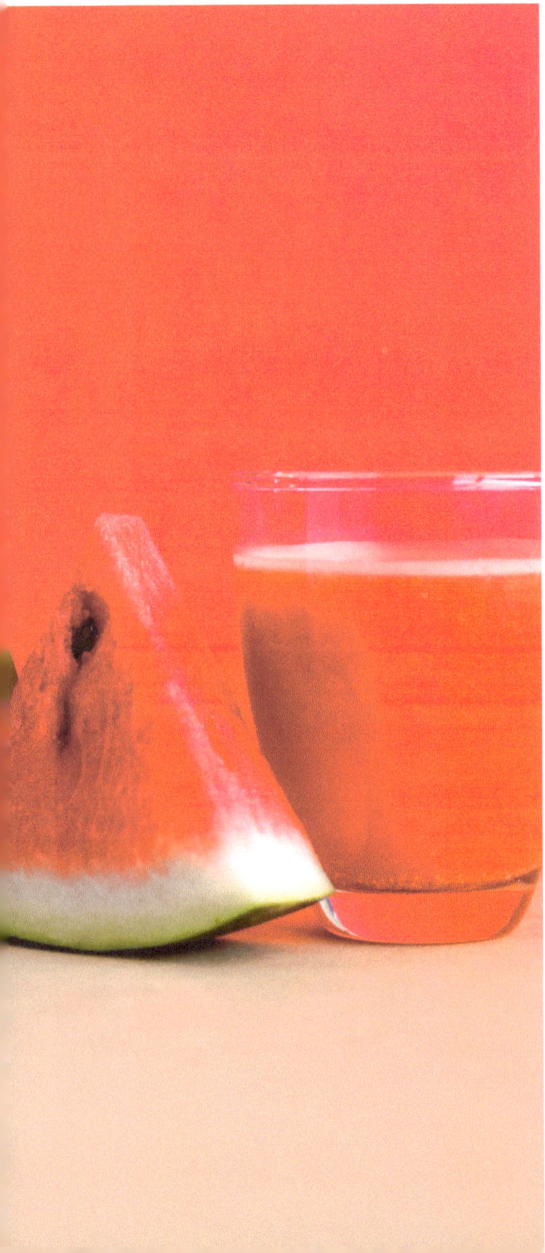

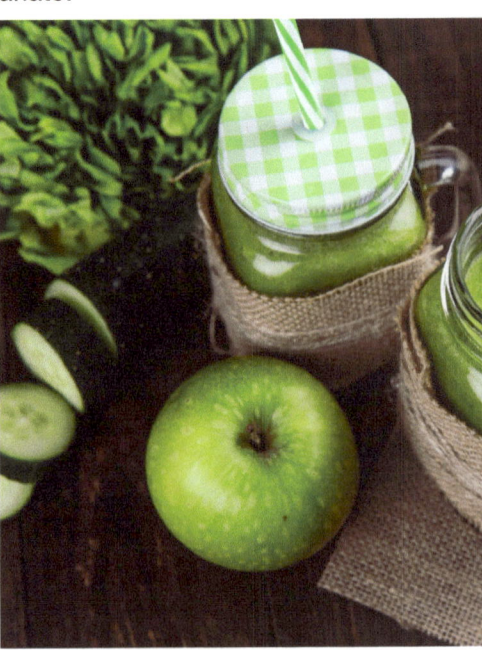

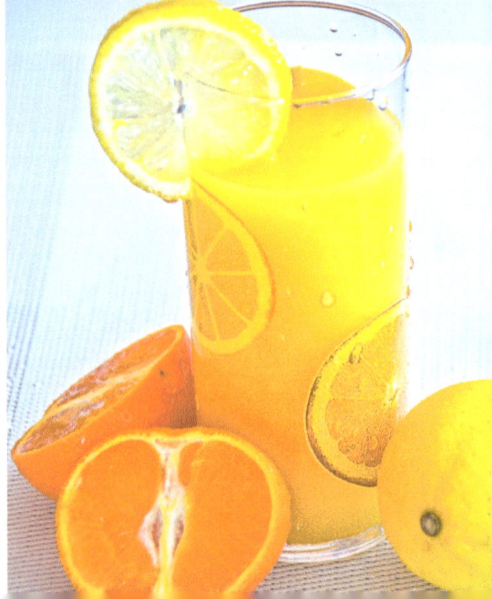

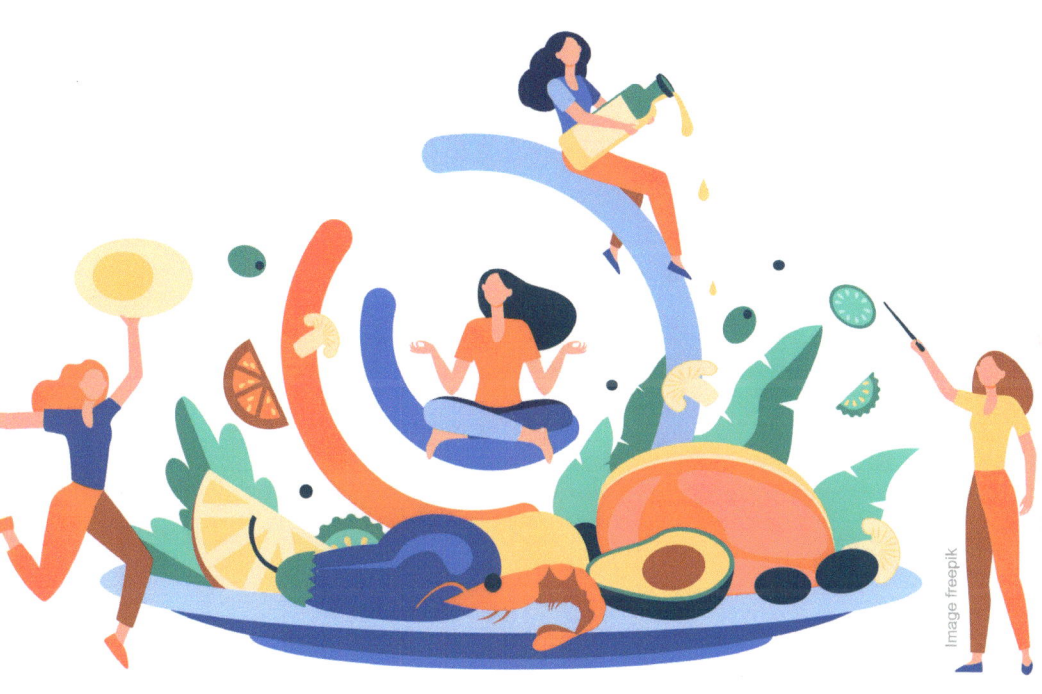

Image freepik

You don't have to cook fancy or complicated masterpieces-just *good* food from *fresh* ingredients.

- Julia Child

Redness... Oiliness... Dryness... Breakouts!

Eeshta Bhatt spent all her teenage years plagued with acne, trying out every cure she could get her hands on, from natural remedies, aloe, tea tree oil, to a variety of antibacterial ointments, gels, oral antibiotics, Japanese skincare for sensitive skin, Korean beauty essentials, acne patches to fruit acid peels.

The quest for perfect glowing skin is never-ending, starting right from your teenage days, or if you're lucky, not until your adult years. It is made even more challenging by the plethora of information you're constantly bombarded with, articles claiming to clear your skin in 1 week, bloggers advertising miraculous serums, facial masks made from anything ranging from honey to potato starch, and products claiming to be miracle workers capable of instantaneously clearing blemishes. This book cuts out all that, aiming to help you achieve healthy, clear skin through advice backed by medical science.

From identifying the causes of your acne and classifying it to planning your meals and treating it, with the help of Dr. Parul Khot, Eeshta guides you through essential steps your skincare routine must include. Through step-by-step tutorials, skincare tips, and advice for choosing cleansers, moisturizers, and more, this book will help you take care of your skin. So even if acne does attack, you're not left scrambling for a remedy, forced to settle for any old cream you can find.

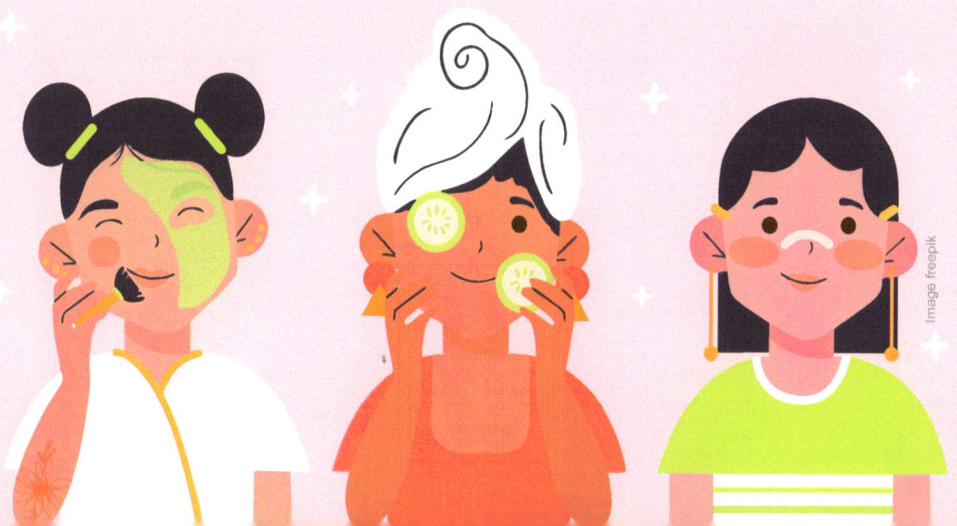

Image freepik

www.ingramcontent.com/pod-product-compliance
Lightning Source LLC
Chambersburg PA
CBHW041059180526
45172CB00001B/35